THE
GLAM
GUIDE

First published in 2015 by
HEADLINE PUBLISHING GROUP

1

Cataloguing in Publication Data is available from the British Library

Designed by Siobhan Hooper
All Photography by Laurie Fletcher except as follows:
    Shutterstock: 12, 25, 29, 44, 90, 112, 125 (right), 201, 205
    Mark Hooper: 164-168, 170-171
Illustrations by Sally Faye
Hair Styling by Gareth Smith

Trade Paperback ISBN 978 1 4722 2840 6

Printed and bound in Germany by Mohn Media

HEADLINE PUBLISHING GROUP
An Hachette UK Company
338 Euston Road
London NW1 3BH

www.headline.co.uk
www.hachette.co.uk

fleur de force

THE
GLAM
GUIDE

headline

Contents

Introduction

When I was a teenager I always wanted to be one of those perfectly groomed girls. You know the kind: not a hair out of place, never-chipped nails and with perfect poise. The older I got, the more I realised I was never going to be like that. I loved beauty and fashion from a young age, used to sew my own dresses for school parties and always had makeup on my Christmas wish list, but I wasn't one of those 'perfect' girls. I was happy to leave the house with no makeup when I felt like it, and enjoyed spending time with my friends and family far more than taking that extra half an hour doing my hair.

When I got to university I had more time on my hands than ever before and discovered a group of girls making videos about beauty and style on YouTube. I quickly became addicted. I started my own YouTube channel to share my thoughts and recommendations, but also to be part of the online community of beauty and fashion lovers that I identified with so strongly. They were glamorous, confident and, most importantly, relatable. My then boyfriend (now husband) Mike didn't believe many people would follow me, but thought it would be a fun hobby and promised he would buy me some new makeup brushes if I reached fifty followers, so I was off . . .

What began as a fun hobby quickly turned into something much bigger. Fifty followers became a hundred, a hundred became a thousand and, more recently, that number unbelievably passed a million. By the time I left university my passion had become my career and I've spent the past five years seeking out the best products, top tips and easiest ways to look more fabulous. I still don't think I'm the most naturally glamorous woman to walk the earth, but I certainly know how to enjoy myself trying to get there. Now, after years of creating content online, and as

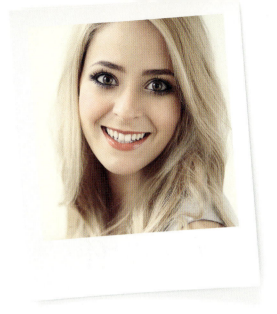

a direct result of the unrelenting support of my YouTube audience, I have been given the chance to put what I've learned into writing.

I've always hated beauty and fashion books that read like rule books because what works for some doesn't work for everyone. This book is a little different, simply offering my advice and tips for living a glam life. To me, being glamorous isn't all about the traditional perception of glamour, or about being 'perfect'. It's about developing your own personal sense of style, discovering what suits you and learning to be fabulous in your own individual way. It's also about learning to treat yourself well – being active and eating a balanced diet to make your skin glow, your hair shine and keep your energy levels pumping so you can feel fantastic both inside and out.

The great thing about YouTube is that you have the ability to ask your audience what they want to learn from you and what matters to them. That's exactly what I did, and this book therefore contains a huge variety of advice, tips and tricks as requested by the people that follow me, whether they're looking for makeup tips, wardrobe cheats or healthy lifestyle motivation. I'm also sharing some of my secrets to becoming successful online, just in case you too want to start your own blog or become a YouTube pro.

Whether you're reading this book having watched my videos for years, or simply picked it up by chance, I hope that you find some of my tips useful and come away feeling inspired and just that little bit more glamorous.

Zoe x

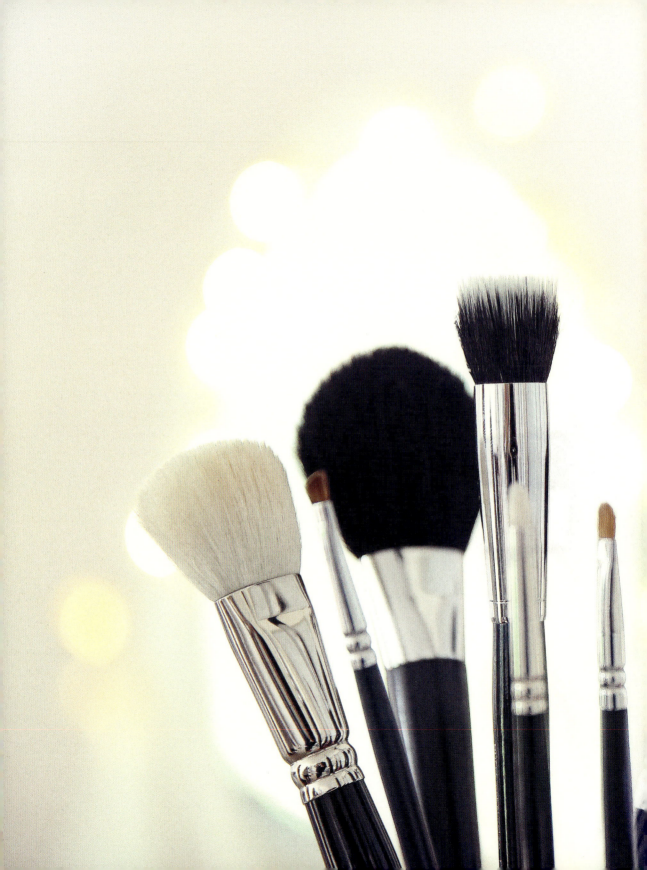

Beauty

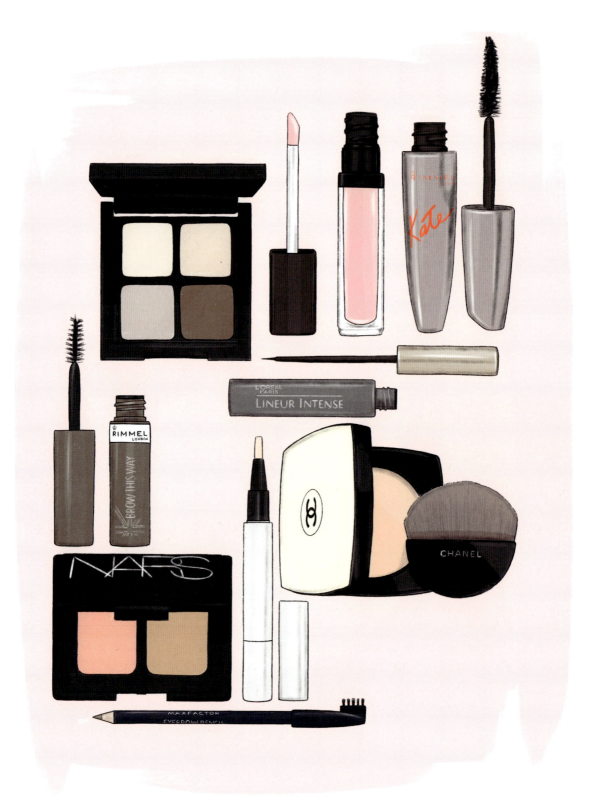

Where to Start

Beauty. The dictionary defines it as 'a combination of qualities such as shape, colour or form that pleases the aesthetic senses, especially the sight'. There are such strict ideas of what qualifies as 'beautiful' these days, it's hard to remember it's all down to individual taste, style and preference. There should be no strict 'rules' in the beauty world. A lot of books like this read like a beauty rule book, telling you what you *must or must not do*. I hate that.

Beauty is individual. Not only because taste differs, but also because everyone's face is different. Some faces can 'take' a lot of makeup, others look ridiculous fully made-up. Trying to be something you're not, or re-creating a beauty look that simply doesn't suit you never looks good, no matter what anyone says about it being the 'right' way to do things. Therefore, my advice is to go with your instincts. Try new things, but only stick to the ones that suit you, and don't let anyone tell you what you should or shouldn't be doing if you're not happy with doing it.

Confidence is the key to real beauty (and style, but we'll get to that later in the book!). Those glowingly beautiful girls you see in life always seem to ooze confidence. Makeup can really help to boost your confidence, but it's all about getting the right balance. Too much can make you feel self-conscious, yet going bare-faced can also leave you feeling insecure.

I often get asked about a 'makeup starter kit', i.e. what people should buy if they are totally new to makeup, or want to give their makeup bag a little overhaul. It's easy to answer with a simple list of products – mascara, concealer, foundation or tinted moisturiser, blusher, bronzer, eyeliner, a basic eye shadow quad and a lipstick or gloss – but not everyone will need all of these items, and some people will want a lot more. Everyone's different, so it's all about working out what you're looking for. I hope the following chapters help you to navigate the world of beauty a little easier, to find out what works for you, and what makes you feel your most confident and beautiful.

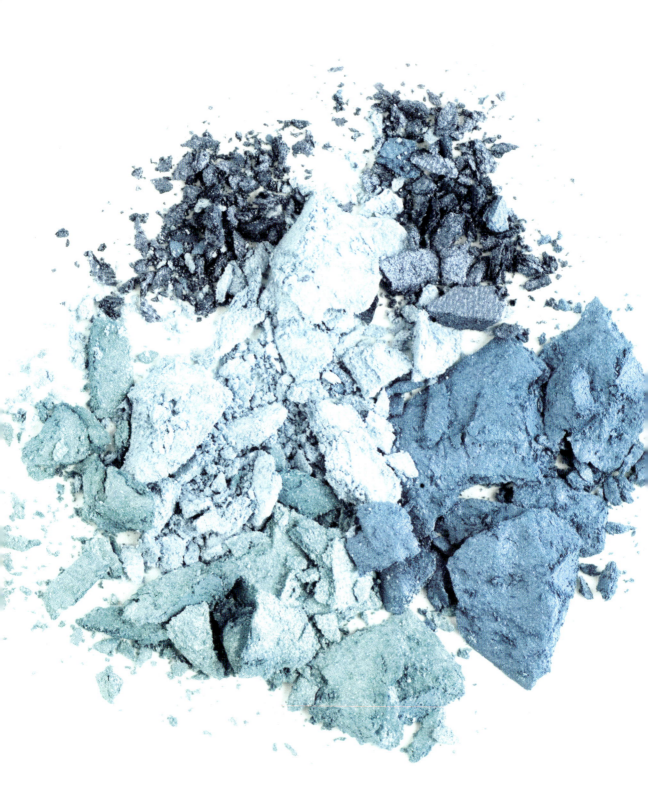

Colour Wheel

Choosing the right shades and tones for your makeup can make a huge difference. You might be applying it like a pro, but if the shade doesn't suit you, it'll never look perfect. The colour wheel has been used by artists and makeup artists alike for ever. It's really simple to use and it will transform the way you think about colour in your makeup, outfits and even in your home.

On a basic level, colours that sit directly opposite each other on the colour wheel are **complementary**, and will make each other stand out and look more vibrant when used together. Similarly, colours that sit next to each other on the colour wheel are **analogous**, which means they will look quietly good together. By pairing analogous colours, you can create depth and mood.

If you're ever stuck in a makeup rut and want to change up your shade, or even decide which accessory to pair with your new favourite dress, the colour wheel can give you a helping hand, and perhaps a little inspiration too!

Using the colour wheel as a basis, below are some of my suggestions for eye makeup based on your eye colour. While eyes are one of the key focal points on your face, especially for makeup, remember that these colour suggestions are also applicable to your other makeup and clothing too. If you don't want to go for a bold makeup look, try a dress in that colour!

BLUE EYES

Make them pop: Go for gold, orange, peach, coral or copper tones.

Accentuate your assets: Bronze or rusty browns that still have an orange tone to them, but aren't so daring.

GREEN EYES

Make them pop: If you're feeling adventurous, go for a vibrant purple or deeper burgundy shade.

Accentuate your assets: For subtler makeup or daytime wear, choose deep olive, sage or green-brown shades.

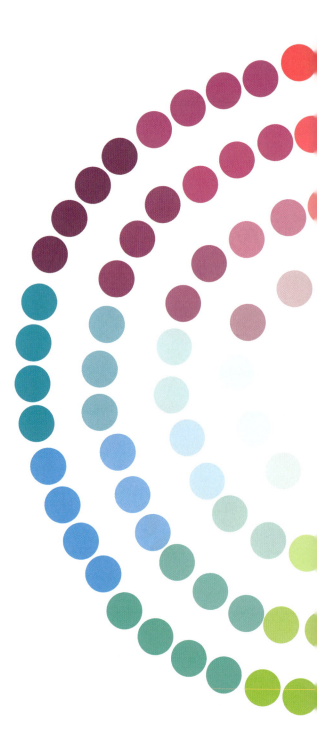

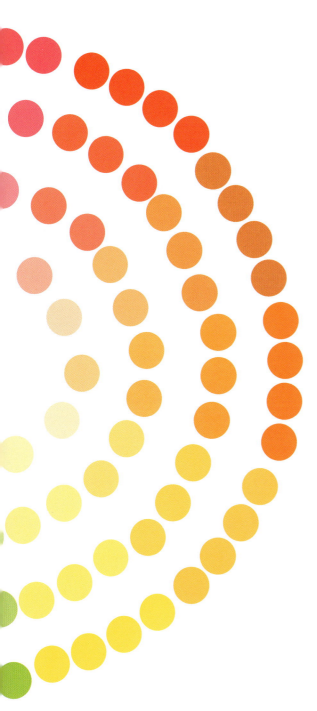

BROWN EYES

Make them pop: Brown eyes suit most shades, but I think they look their best when paired with metallics. Add a beautiful metallic accent to your classic smokey eye to really enhance your brown eyes.

Accentuate your assets: My favourite, subtler look for brown eyes is to stick with simple, neutral matte eye shadows and a classic liquid liner. This never goes out of style and looks particularly alluring on dark eyes.

GREY EYES

Make them pop: Choose metallic silver to really accentuate your pale grey eyes. This looks particularly good when used as an accent with a deep black smokey eye. This will work in the same way if you have green-grey or blue-grey eyes.

Accentuate your assets: Choose cooler-toned neutrals like taupe, grey or silver.

Makeup Brushes

There are so many makeup brushes available, it's hard to know which ones are essential. If you choose the right brushes and take care of them well, they can last you for many years. So which ones do you really need in your makeup bag?

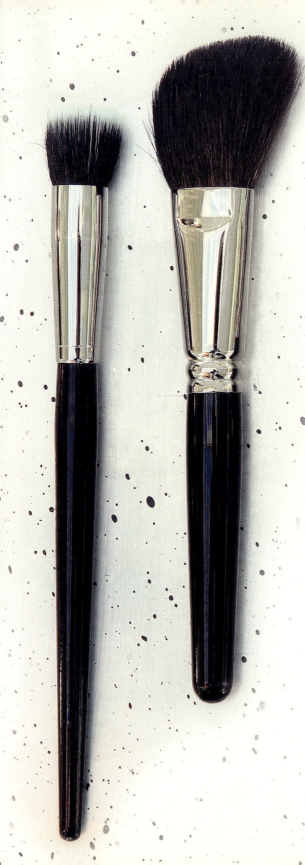

FOUNDATION

There are lots of different shapes and sizes, but my favourites are small flat-top brushes you can use to really buff the product into your skin. They give you a really natural, polished look.

CONTOUR, BRONZER AND HIGHLIGHTER

You might want different brushes for each of the above, but you can use the same one and clean it in between applications. I use angled fluffy brushes for contouring, bronzing and highlighting, as they are perfectly shaped to fit the contours of your face and make application more precise.

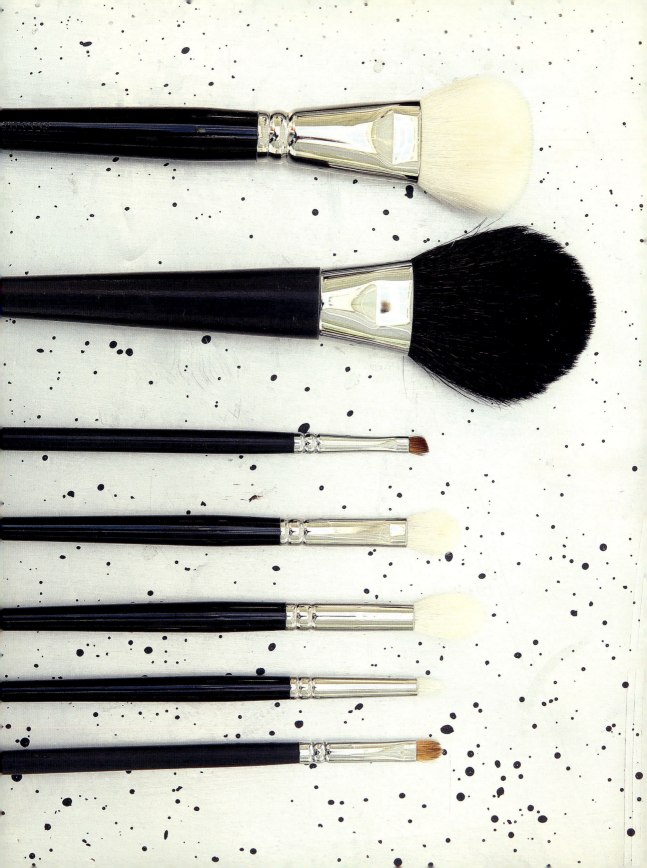

BLUSHER

While a lot of people are tempted to use huge powder brushes for blusher, it's actually better to go for a smaller one, so you have more control over application. Too much blusher is never a good look!

POWDER

A large fluffy brush is perfect for applying and blending in powder. Make sure you choose one with super-soft bristles, so you can powder without shifting any of your other makeup.

SMALL ANGLED BRUSH

A small, angled brush is a great addition to your makeup bag as you can use it with a matte eye shadow to fill in your brows, or you can use it to line your lash line with eye shadow.

BASIC EYE SHADOW

My favourite brush for applying eye shadow is the MAC 217, or similar. These are fluffy but slightly flat, so you can use them for both base application and for blending.

EYE SHADOW BLENDING

A larger fluffy, domed brush is perfect for blending out darker shades or harsh lines in your eye shadow. Make sure you clean it every time to make blending totally foolproof!

EYELINER

Not totally essential, but very useful! If you like your eyeliner to look a little smudgy, choose a small, pointed pencil brush to blend darker colours along your lash line in a fraction of the time. You can also use this to apply powder over gel liner to set it, smudge kohl liner or apply powder shadow under your lower lashes for definition.

LIPS

A lip brush is useful if you like to wear a bold lip. It allows you to apply your lipstick more precisely, and a portable one with a lid is even better, as it can be thrown into your handbag and used for on-the-go touch-ups.

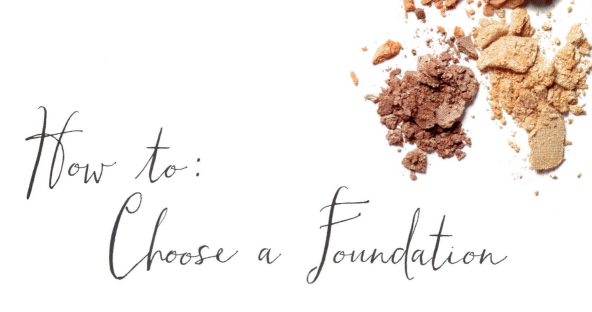

How to: Choose a Foundation

A good foundation has the ability to hide a multitude of imperfections, giving you a perfect, glowing complexion and boosting your confidence at the same time. A bad one, however, can leave your skin looking cakey, orange or ghostly pale, and anything but natural. Finding the perfect formulation, shade and means of application can seem daunting, but it's worth spending a little extra time to find your ideal match. Follow my simple guide below to find the perfect foundation for you.

FORMULATION

When looking for your perfect base, finding the right formulation can be as important as picking the correct shade. If you have oily skin, look for formulas that are oil-free, claim to control oil or give a matte finish. Those with dry skin should look for hydrating, moisture-rich, 'dewy' formulas. Most foundations will be labelled accordingly, but if you're struggling, try the formula out with your fingers. You'll be able to feel the texture, and see the finish for yourself. If you have combination or normal skin you have a bit more choice. Decide what finish you like the look of the most and go from there.

COVERAGE

The type of coverage is usually down to personal preference, but can also be seasonal. Most people tend to go for a lighter foundation in the summer and a thicker, creamier, higher-coverage foundation in the winter. If you want a high coverage foundation, thicker liquids and creams are your best bet. For lighter, more natural coverage, tinted moisturisers, BB creams or thinner liquid formulas are great.

SHADE: WARM, COOL OR NEUTRAL?

Determining whether or not you have a warm (yellow), cool (pink) or neutral undertone to your skin can help you choose the right foundation shade, but it can be confusing, especially if you have an uneven skin tone. In natural light, look at the veins on the inside of your wrist. If they look blue, you have cool undertones; if they look green, you have warm undertones; and if it's hard to tell, you probably have a neutral skin tone. To double-check, take a look at which items of clothing and jewellery flatter you the most. If you lean towards blue or purple clothing and silver jewellery, you are cool, and if you suit yellow or orange clothing and gold jewellery, then you are warm. If you can't notice too much of a difference in what colours suit you, you're probably neutral.

SPF

SPF is a bit of a love/hate thing when it comes to foundation. A lot of people worry that SPF can result in ghostly-looking 'flashback' in photographs. If you're buying a foundation for nights out, or if you're going to be photographed a lot, it's advisable to stick to a foundation with little or no SPF. For everyday use, it's great to have an SPF in your foundation for extra protection, but I usually supplement it with a separate sunscreen to prevent premature ageing.

TIPS FOR FINDING YOUR PERFECT MATCH

- Testing foundation on the back of your hand won't give you the perfect match, as your hands are usually a few shades darker than your face. Instead, test foundation at the back of your jawline (next to your ear) to get the perfect match. This area tends to give you a good representation of your natural skin tone, as it's not an area prone to discolouration or redness.

- Ask a friend or shop attendant to help you choose the best shade, if you can, and make sure you get outside and see what your skin looks like in natural light.

- If you can get a sample, try before you buy! This is the best way to give foundation a proper trial run before you invest. If you do manage to get your hands on a sample, apply it in the morning and give it a full test-run to see if it gives you the coverage, finish and wear-time that you're looking for. If you're shopping in a department store, it's always worth asking for a small sample. Most high-end brands will be happy to give you a small pot to try at home.

- Shopping online for foundation is very risky, so avoid this at all costs unless you already know your shade.

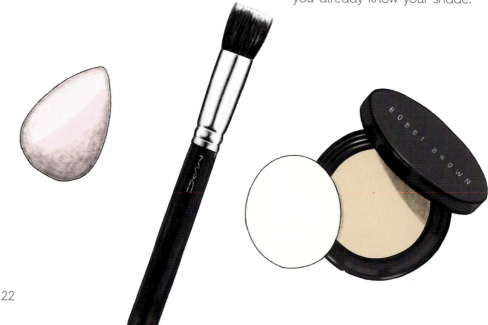

APPLICATION

Primer

Foundation primer has become really popular over the past few years. It usually comes in the form of a clear, translucent white or beige cream that smoothes and perfects the surface of the skin before you apply your foundation, making it look smoother and last for longer. However, it's not always an essential step. If you have oily skin, large pores or want your foundation to last especially long that day, it's definitely worth investing in, but if your foundation lasts well anyway, don't feel you need to apply primer beforehand.

Tools

Everyone has a different preference when it comes to application. Personally, I prefer small, flat-top brushes to really buff my foundation into my skin. Traditional flat foundation brushes work best with liquid foundations. If you like using sponges, make sure you replace them regularly. Domed or egg-shaped sponges like the Beauty Blender work really well, especially when you dampen them with clean water before use. Many of the world's best makeup artists swear by using hands to apply foundation, as it helps to warm the product and therefore it will blend into the skin better, but it's always different for each person and each foundation.

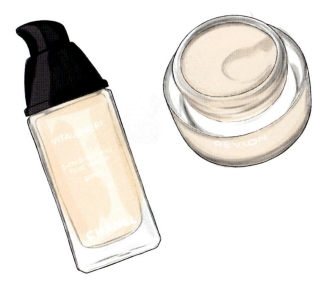

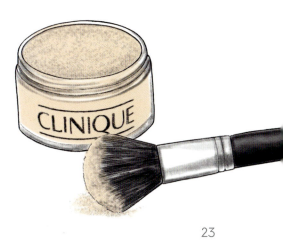

Concealer 101

Choosing the right concealer depends on what you're trying to cover up. A lot of people use one concealer for all the different imperfections on their face, which is fine if you have no major discolouration. If you're trying to cover up more pronounced redness or darker imperfections, however, it's worth investing in a couple of different shades, as you'll get much better results.

DARK CIRCLES

If you have dark under-eye circles, go for a salmon pink concealer (Bobbi Brown and Laura Mercier both make brilliant ones). The orange tone in the product will help to balance out the purple and blue tones under your eyes, and the pink tone will help to brighten the area, making you look more awake. This also works for dark spots.

REDNESS

If you're covering up redness or spots, you need to go for a green-toned concealer or a yellow-green shade, which will neutralise redness. Some colour-correcting products are simply green. These look pretty scary, and for most cases may be a little more than you need, but if you want to use a green corrector shade, then make sure you only use a tiny bit, exactly where you need it. Also remember to pop a tiny bit of flesh-toned concealer over the top afterwards, to even out the skin tone around the problem area, and to make sure you can't see any green! Avon make a great colour-correcting palette and Bobbi Brown also do great correctors of all tones that you can mix and match as you require.

Tip: It's a common misconception that YSL's iconic Touche Éclat is a concealer. It's actually a highlighter, and should be used as one to avoid highlighting your imperfections instead of concealing them! See page 39 on highlighting to find out how.

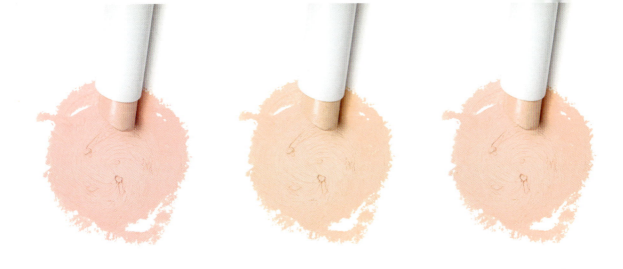

APPLICATION

When to Apply

There is quite a debate in the makeup world over when to apply your concealer – before or after foundation? It's all down to individual preference. I personally prefer to apply it after my foundation, so I don't move the concealer out of place, or blend it across my face into the wrong area.

Where to Apply

To avoid applying too much, especially to blemishes, dot on concealer only where you need it and not in the surrounding area, as that is where you'll blend the product in to make it look natural. For your under-eye area, apply concealer in a triangle shape (with your bottom lash line being one side of the triangle). This will make sure you're applying the product where you need it and it doesn't stray to the outer corner of your eye, where it tends to look cakey.

How to Apply

I prefer to blend concealer in with my fingers (as it warms the product) or use a slightly damp makeup sponge. The latter will stop your concealer looking cakey and is especially good for under the eyes.

Don't Forget to Set!

To keep your concealer in place for longer, make sure you give it a light dusting with translucent powder after application. You should do this to your entire face, as you want to set your foundation too. It will reduce the need for touch-ups throughout the day.

Tip: Choose a concealer one shade lighter than you think you need, as it tends to dry slightly darker than it looks in the tube. Don't go too light though, as you don't want to highlight and draw attention to any problem areas you are trying to conceal.

All About Brows

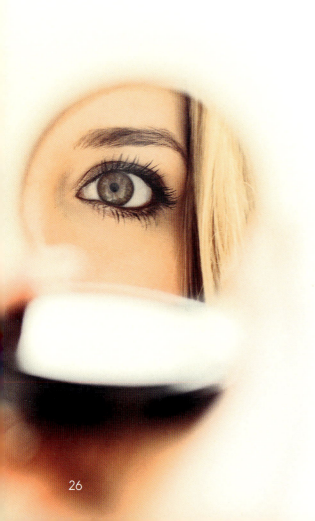

Even though I've been a makeup obsessive for many years, brows were quite a mystery to me until fairly recently. Many people just get by plucking any stray hairs, but properly grooming your eyebrows can make such a difference to your look, and is well worth taking the time to do. Well-defined brows can help to enhance the other features on your face, making you look more polished, youthful and well-groomed, even with no makeup on. Here are my tips for getting to grips with your brows.

FIND THE RIGHT SHAPE

The 'perfect' brow should be in line with your nose, and directly diagonal from the bottom of your nose and the outer corner of your eye (see diagram). In terms of shape, it's always best to enhance what you've got rather than change it. Over-plucking is the biggest mistake, as it can take years to grow back.

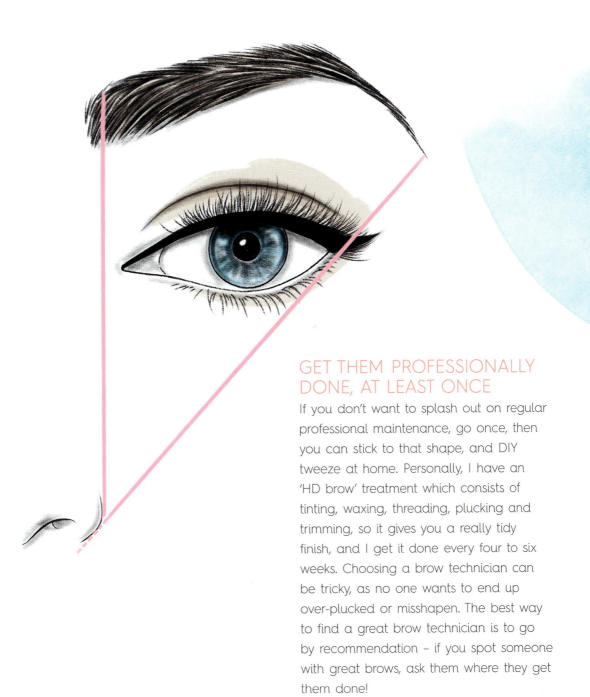

GET THEM PROFESSIONALLY DONE, AT LEAST ONCE

If you don't want to splash out on regular professional maintenance, go once, then you can stick to that shape, and DIY tweeze at home. Personally, I have an 'HD brow' treatment which consists of tinting, waxing, threading, plucking and trimming, so it gives you a really tidy finish, and I get it done every four to six weeks. Choosing a brow technician can be tricky, as no one wants to end up over-plucked or misshapen. The best way to find a great brow technician is to go by recommendation – if you spot someone with great brows, ask them where they get them done!

PICK THE RIGHT BROW MAKEUP FOR YOUR NEEDS

Powder, pencil, liquid or mascara? Deciding on the right makeup for your brows can be tricky. Some of you won't need it, or might need it on just one brow. (I have one brow that is practically perfect, yet the other is patchy and needs a little help!)

- The easiest makeup to fill in your brows is **powder**. Used with an angled brush, it's quick and foolproof. You can also use a matte eye shadow shade. My favourite powder is from MAC, but Rimmel also make an affordable duo option.
- **Pencils** are the most convenient and portable, but also make it easier to fill your brows in a little too heavily. Once you get the hang of them, however, pencils are the quickest and most travel-friendly option. My favourite brow pencils are from Tom Ford and Max Factor.

- Some brands make liquid, felt-tip **brow pens**. These are a great long-lasting option, but are probably the hardest to perfect.
- If you suffer from thinning or sparse brows as opposed to patchiness, then **brow mascara** is the best option. Benefit makes a great one and Rimmel also do a more affordable version. It sounds scary, but you simply brush it into your brows to thicken them up – just make sure there isn't too much product on the brush!

NO MATTER WHAT YOU GO FOR, YOU WANT TO APPLY IT IN SHORT, LIGHT STROKES.

This emulates your natural hairs and will look the most natural.

COMB AND SET!

Once you're happy with your look, blend in any colour and set it in place using a clear brow gel or brow comb and wax. Brush upwards and outwards to keep the brows looking lifted and neat.

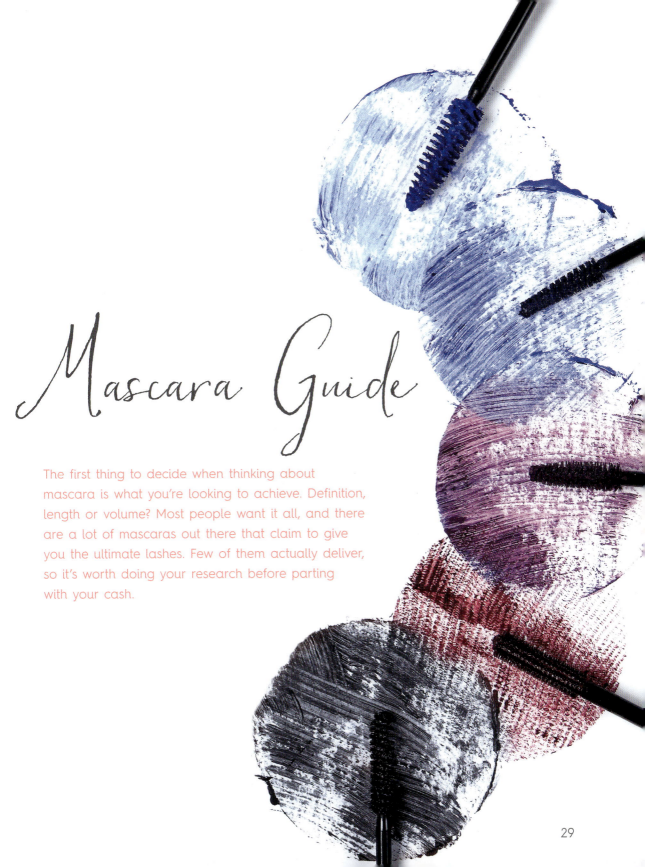

Mascara Guide

The first thing to decide when thinking about mascara is what you're looking to achieve. Definition, length or volume? Most people want it all, and there are a lot of mascaras out there that claim to give you the ultimate lashes. Few of them actually deliver, so it's worth doing your research before parting with your cash.

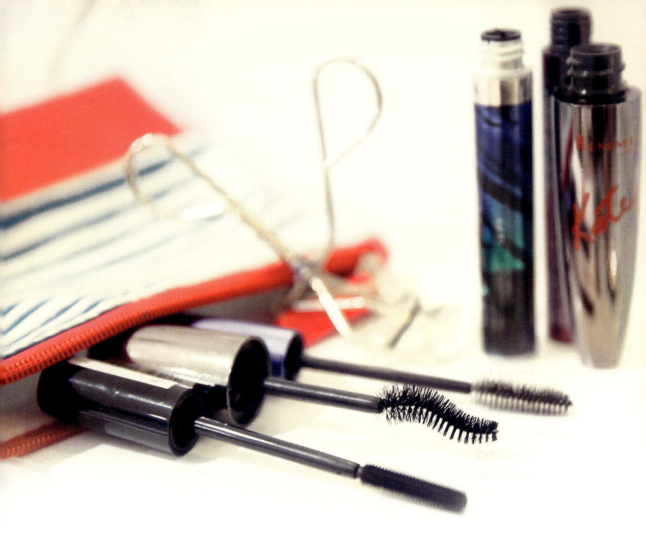

BRUSH

The shape and type of brush makes a big difference to the end result. Rubber brushes with lots of fine bristles tend to be the best for definition. Natural brushes tend to give you a more fluttery, natural finish. Unusual brush shapes (twisted, round, wavy) may seem gimmicky, but a lot of them actually do work! I always look up several reviews online before deciding whether or not to buy a new mascara. To find the best reviews, I simply Google the product itself and look for professional, blog or video reviews of the product. If I see a blogger I already know and trust reviewing a product, I'll take their word for it, otherwise I look up three or four different opinions before making my decision.

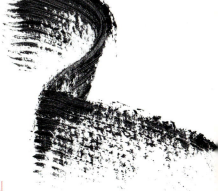

CURL

If you have very short or straight lashes, it's well worth investing in an eyelash curler. These have been around for years and years. If you're not already a convert, once you use one, it's hard to go without! Even if you don't use mascara, curling your lashes can help to open up your eyes, making you look more awake and your lashes appear longer. Shu Uemura make the best out there. Their eyelash curler is a world-renowned cult beauty buy.

HOW TO CURL YOUR LASHES

- Curl your lashes before you apply mascara.
- Start at the root of the lashes.
- Apply pressure in short pulses for around five seconds.
- Repeat halfway along the length of the lash for maximum impact.

APPLICATION

It may seem obvious, but there are a few tips for applying your mascara that can make a big difference!

- Tilt your head back when applying to the upper lashes, and forward for the lower lashes. This will help you to avoid getting mascara on your eyelids.
- Don't 'pump' the wand! This only introduces air (and bacteria) into your mascara tube. Twist your mascara around in its tube before applying. This way, you'll get more product on the wand, but your mascara won't dry out so quickly and you'll be less likely to have a family of bacteria growing in your mascara tube!
- Start at the root and 'wiggle' the wand from side to side as you coat your lashes. Wait for the first coat to partially dry before you apply the next (do your other eye in the meantime).
- Remove any mistakes with a dry cotton bud (using a wet one will remove any other makeup you've already applied) only once your mascara is totally dry, so it won't smudge.

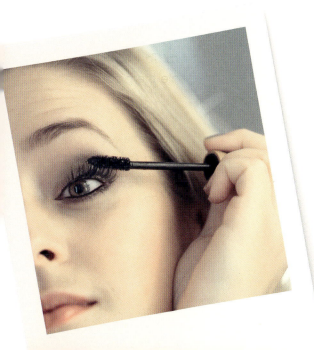

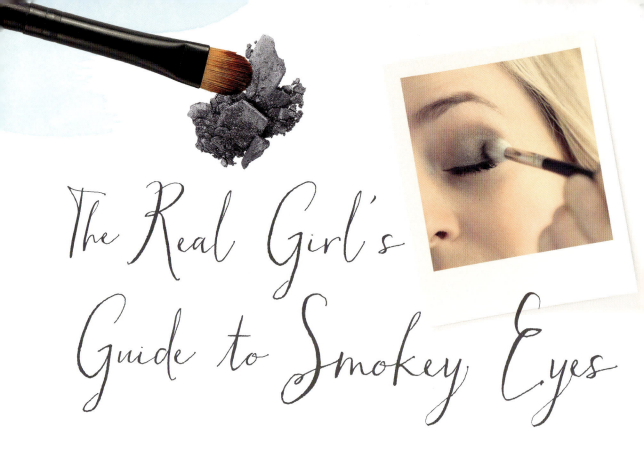

The Real Girl's Guide to Smokey Eyes

There are thousands of video tutorials on YouTube showing you how to achieve the 'perfect' smokey eye. But without a lot of practice, smokey eyes can still be tricky! Here are my tips for getting the perfect smokey eye, even if you're a makeup novice . . .

THE STICKY TAPE TRICK

If you struggle to keep your eye shadow where you want it, and often end up with dark fallout underneath your eyes, use a little bit of Sellotape or a Post-it note. Line it up with your lower lashes, stick it on, apply your eye shadow, remove it carefully when you're done, and you'll have a perfect, neat line! If you choose Sellotape, make sure you stick it on your arm or clothing a couple of times to reduce the stickiness before applying it to your delicate eye area.

START OFF SMALL

A full-on smokey eye can be daunting, and doesn't suit everyone. You can start by using your eyeliner to create a more subtle version. Apply a rough line along your upper lashes and use a blending brush to soften it out. Repeat this a couple of times.

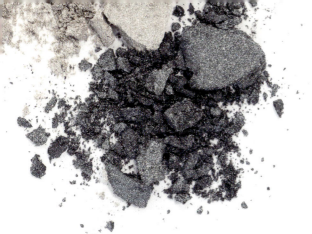

DON'T FORGET TO BLEND!

Blending is the hardest and most laborious part of creating a smokey eye, and is often where people go wrong. Make sure your brushes are totally clean before you start and have one brush for applying the eye shadow and another for blending. Apply a light flesh-tone matte eye shadow all over your lids, up to your brows, before you start. This will give you a good base and something to blend the darker colour in to. If you're struggling, choose a slightly darker matte shade and use it with a fluffy domed brush to help blend the darker eye shadow more easily.

ADD A LITTLE COLOUR

Some people think that smokey eyes always have to be black, but if black is too harsh for you, go for something softer, like a warm brown. You can still get the sultry, smokey effect, but it's easier to pull off and you can wear it in the daytime too. It's also nice to inject a little colour or sparkle by adding a shimmery eye shadow to the centre of your eyelid (where your pupil would be when your eyes are open) and blending it out across your eyelid.

KEEP YOUR LIPS NEUTRAL

Bright lips with smokey eyes nearly always look OTT! Choose a nude, or neutral pink lip colour to perfectly complement your smokey eye.

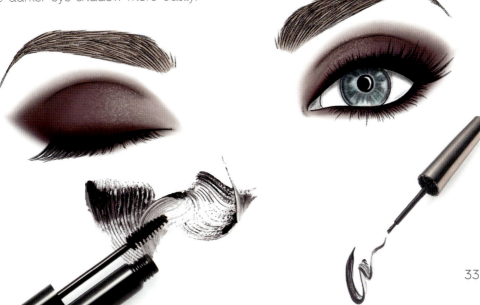

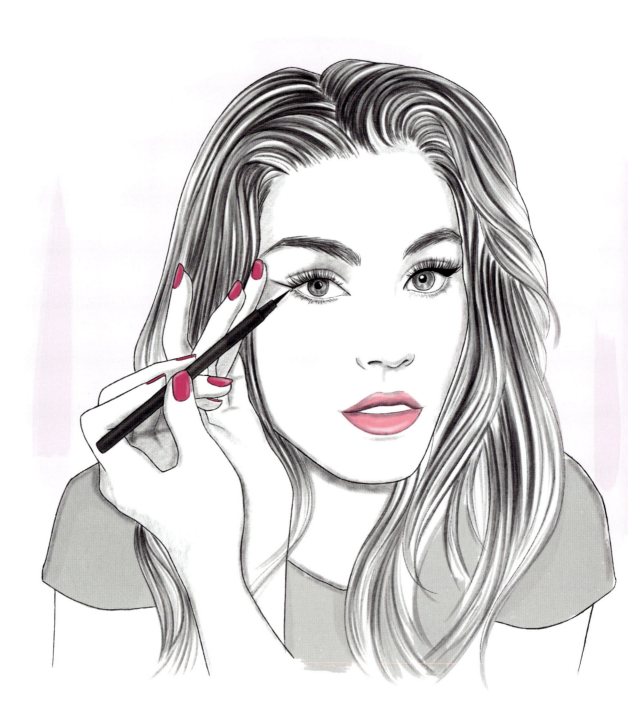

Liquid Liner

Eyeliner is a fantastic way to both define your eyes and to create the illusion of a different shape. While pencil or gel eye liner may be easier to master, there is something about the simple sophistication of perfectly applied liquid liner that makes it something every girl should learn how to do at some point in her life.

It took me a while to master liquid liner, and to find the few products that really work for me, but now I've perfected it, I wear it all the time, as it's a quick and easy way to look polished in just a couple of minutes.

CHOOSE THE RIGHT PRODUCT

It can be tricky to know which eyeliners are the best, because without trying them out yourself, you can't tell what will glide on easily, stay black and last all day. Look up reviews online for recommendations from people who have actually tried and tested the products. My favourites are from Burberry, MAC, NYX and L'Oréal Paris.

APPLICATION

Start from the inner corner and draw a rough, thin line all the way along your lashes. When you reach the outer corner, flip your pen or brush around and draw on a small flick that lines up with your lower lash line – this bit's important, as the right shape of flick is different for every eye, so make sure you use your own eye shape for guidance. Then you can go back over the line, making it wider and smoother until you have the desired look. Apply your eye shadow first, and your mascara after. If you make any mistakes, especially with the flick, it's usually quicker and easier (depending on how much eye shadow you have on!) to remove the whole line and start again.

PRACTICE MAKES PERFECT!

Using liquid liner is one of those annoying things where practice really does make perfect. The more you do it, the better you'll get!

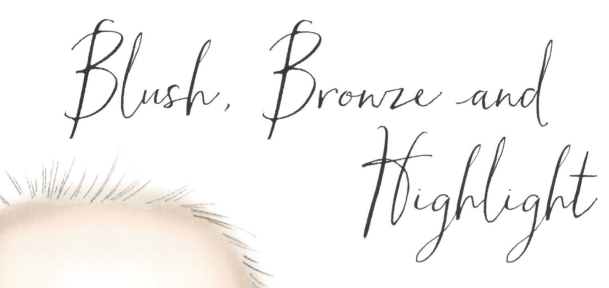

Blush, Bronze and Highlight

Whilst most women have at least one blusher or bronzer and perhaps a highlighter in their makeup bag, a lot of people aren't using them to their full potential. Blushers, bronzers and highlighters are best used together, to enhance your features to their maximum potential. Here are my tips for choosing the right shade and formula, and how to apply all three to make the most of your makeup without overdoing it.

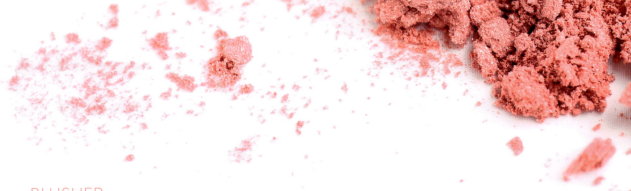

BLUSHER

Shade

Choosing the perfect shade of blusher for you depends on your natural colouring, so it's worth thinking about your natural skin tone and eye colour. Warmer, more yellow-toned blushers will suit those with warm, yellow undertones, and cooler shades with hints of purple or blue will suit cool skin tones. If it's something you want to wear every day, you might not want to go for a colour with a lot of shimmer or something really bright, but if you want to have a bit more fun with your makeup, a bright blusher is a great way to do that and there are so many options out there!

Formulation

Whether you choose a powder, cream, gel or liquid formula depends on personal preference. I prefer powders, as they generally last for longer and are easier to apply over any formula of foundation.

Cream and gel formulas are great for the summertime, but I personally don't like liquids, as they usually dry really quickly and give you limited blending time.

Application

Apply blusher to the apples of your cheeks and blend it outwards and upwards in line with your cheekbone. Try to keep blusher at least two fingers in distance away from your nose and eyes, to keep it looking natural. Use a smaller brush to ensure accuracy with your application. It's easy to apply too much blusher, so start with a little, blend it out, then apply more if needed.

Tip: If you apply too much blusher, use a little face powder on a clean brush and blend it over the top, to tone down the colour.

BRONZER

Shade

The shade of bronzer you choose depends on what you want to use it for. While some people only use bronzer to warm their complexion and give the illusion of a tan, others use it for 'contouring', cleverly sculpting and defining their features. For creating a sun-kissed effect, you can get away with a warmer, more orange-toned bronzer with a slight shimmer to it. It's important that you don't go too orange, or too shimmery, as you don't want to look like an Oompa-Loompa, but in moderation this can look really pretty. If you want to use your bronzer for contouring, go for a slightly cooler shade with no shimmer, avoiding anything with orange or yellow undertones.

Formulation

Powder is the most common, but you can also get cream and gel bronzers. Wet formulations are often less forgiving and have higher levels of pigmentation, so if you're not very confident, or want to be able to apply your bronzer quickly in the morning, go for a powder.

Application

As with shade, how you apply your bronzer depends on the look you want to go for. If you want a sun-kissed look, apply your bronzer where the sun would naturally hit your face: along your cheekbones and jawline and on your forehead, using what remains on your brush down the centre of your nose. If you want a contoured look that will make your face appear slimmer and define your natural facial features, apply your bronzer to the hollows of your cheeks, on your temples (blending it up onto the forehead) and under your jawline. You can also take it a step further by applying your contour colour along the sides of your nose to make it appear narrower, but make sure you use a smaller brush for this (an eyeshadow-blending brush works really well) as a face brush will be too big and not precise enough.

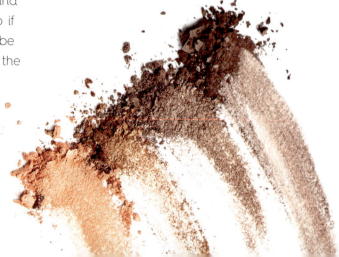

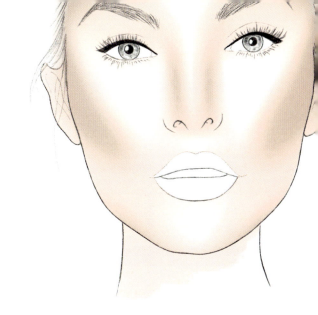

HIGHLIGHTER

Although not as widely used as blushers and bronzers, highlighters are products that draw light and attention to an area of the face, highlighting a specific feature. They can be used to give the skin a natural glow or in conjunction with a contouring powder to provide further contrast, helping define your facial features even more prominently.

Shade

Choosing the right shade of highlighter depends on how subtle you want it to look. For the most subtle effect, choose something that is close to your skin tone. For something more dramatic, you can go for a gold, rose or silver-toned highlighter. I like to avoid any heavy glitter or overtly metallic highlighters, as I don't think they look as good as the subtle glow you can create with more neutral choices. My all-time favourite is Candlelight from Kevyn Aucoin. It manages to create a stunning glow without a fleck of glitter in sight! If you want to contour your features heavily, you're better off highlighting with a light-coloured concealer, as you don't want to overload your face with shimmer.

Formulation

Again, highlighters commonly come in powder, cream and liquid formulas. I like powders, but that's a personal preference. For contouring, you might prefer a cream, which is easier to blend into the skin and often comes without shimmer.

Application

After you've applied your blusher and bronzer, apply highlighter to the high points of your face: on your cheekbones, brow bones, cupid's bow and down the bridge of your nose. If you are using a shimmery formula, it's best to stick to just your cheekbones to avoid a glitterball effect! If you're contouring, applying your highlighter at the opposite points to your contour shade creates the biggest contrast, and therefore the most dramatic results. Extend your contour areas to include between your eyebrows and the centre of your forehead and chin.

Red Lip Tips

No other makeup can transform your look quite like the perfect bold lip. Whether you prefer a classic red, vibrant fuchsia or gothic berry, here are my tips for getting the perfect bold lip every time, and for making it last. If you're struggling to choose the perfect colour, look back to my chapter on the colour wheel. If you don't feel brave enough to go for a really bold shade, but still want to make a statement, opt for something more neutral but at least two shades darker or brighter than your natural lip colour.

PRIME

Make sure your lips are in tip-top condition before applying lipstick, especially matte formulas and darker shades, which can be very unforgiving on dry or cracked lips. Use a soft-bristled toothbrush or a lip scrub to remove any dry skin, then smooth on your favourite lip balm before you start applying your makeup. By the time you come to apply your lipstick, the balm will have absorbed into your lips, leaving them smooth and soft. This will help you to apply your lipstick more smoothly, but also makes it last longer, without any flaking or dryness.

Tip: Making your own lip scrub at home is really easy! Simply mix a little brown sugar with a tiny amount of olive oil or coconut oil. You can make just enough for one use, or put some in a little pot and keep it in your bathroom for future use.

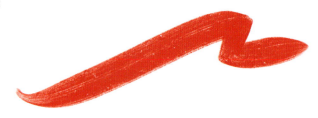

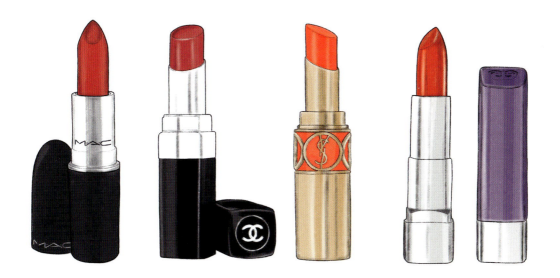

LINE AND DEFINE

To ensure your lipstick stands out to its full potential, simply blend your foundation onto your lips when you're applying your makeup. This creates more of a contrast between your skin and lipstick colour. If you want to use a lip liner to define the shape of your lips, use it to fill in the whole lip. This will act as a base coat, helping your lipstick last for longer.

Tip: You can also use a concealer pencil to further define the lip line after you've applied your lipstick. This works especially well for helping to highlight your cupid's bow.

THE PERFECT FINISH

Apply a generous first coat of lipstick, then use a tissue to carefully blot off any excess colour. Once you've done this, apply a second coat of lipstick. Layering your lip colour will help it last longer, and you'll get a richer, more even covering. Depending on the finish you like, you can also add a gloss over the top. To make your lips look fuller, apply gloss to the centre of your lips and dab it to blend outwards.

Tip: If your lipstick breaks, don't throw it away! Use a lighter to melt the bottom of the broken lipstick bullet, then stick it back into its base, twist it down into the tube and pop it into the fridge for a couple of hours. It'll be almost as good as new!

The Perfect Manicure

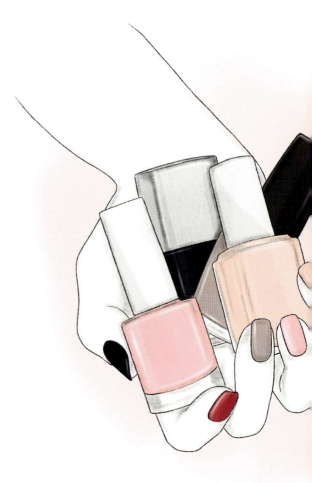

I love the look of perfectly manicured nails, but getting them done professionally can be very expensive and takes an hour out of your day. Here are my top tips for perfecting the art of the at-home manicure, so you can save yourself both time and money.

CLEAN

Remove any old polish from your nails, then wash your hands and give your nails a good scrub to remove any dirt or residue.

BUFF

If your nails are flaky, uneven or ridged (common in toenails!) invest in a four-sided buffer to smooth out the surface of the nail. This will allow you to get a perfectly smooth finish.

FILE

Make sure the length of each nail is the same. Use a nail file to get rid of any sharp edges and chips and then shape your nails into your favourite style.

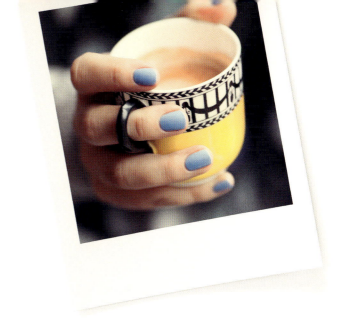

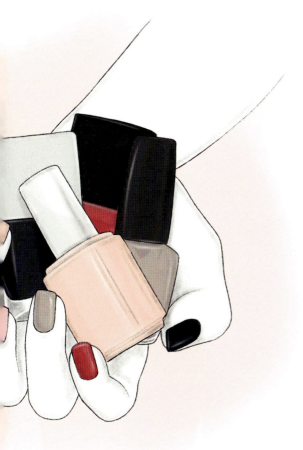

TIDY

Cuticles are something that often get forgotten in DIY manicures, but they make a big difference when you're trying to get the perfect finish. Use a cuticle gel, cream, balm or oil and massage it into your cuticles. When the cuticle skin is soft, push the cuticle back using the flat side of a cuticle (or 'orange') stick. If you have very large cuticles, you may want to trim them using a cuticle trimmer or clipper, but avoid this if you can, as it is easy to damage the skin, leaving it open to infection and soreness.

WASH AND DRY

Wash your hands again to make sure the nail surface is free from any product or residue from filing. Then make sure your nails and hands are completely dry.

BASE COAT

Apply an even layer of your favourite base coat (mine is OPI's Start to Finish, as it can be used as a top coat too). I like to do one streak in the middle, then one on either side, to get even coverage on the nail. Using a base coat is important, as it not only makes your polish look smoother, but will also help to stop the coloured polish from staining your nails.

POLISH

Using the same three-stroke technique as above, apply your polish. If the colour isn't very opaque, resist the temptation to apply it thickly, as this will result in a gloopy finish that takes forever to dry. Applying three or four very thin coats will work much better than two thick ones! Work all the way across your ten nails before returning to the first to apply a second coat. I've found this to be the perfect amount of time to leave the first coat to dry enough.

TOP COAT

Apply a thick layer of your favourite top coat while your polish is still a little wet. This not only helps prevent chipping, but some top coats also make your polish dry faster!

CLEAN UP

If you get polish around your cuticles, a tiny paintbrush dipped in nail polish remover is the best way to remove it. The smaller the brush, the better!

PRACTICE!

Whenever people ask me how I apply my nail polish so smoothly, the answer is always practice, practice, practice! You're not going to be able to do it perfectly first time, but if you follow the above steps, your DIY manicures will be looking salon-worthy in no time!

Tip: When it comes to choosing nail polish, most people buy based on colour, which is unavoidable when it comes to unique shades. But if you're buying classic colours that you're likely to wear a lot, it's worth thinking about which formulas last the longest and apply the smoothest. I love Barry M, Essie and OPI.

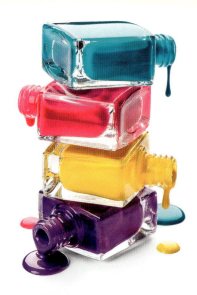

Introduction to Skincare

Some of the most common questions I get asked are: 'Which moisturiser is the best?' and 'What skincare should I be using?' I find it nearly impossible to answer these without having an hour-long conversation with that person, because skincare is totally individual. Everyone's skin is different, so I'm not going to write a list of what you *must* do, or *must* buy, or what you have to *stop* doing, because what works for some doesn't work for others. Instead, I'm going to give you some general advice on how to choose skincare and a basic rundown of what everything does. I hope it helps you to navigate the confusing world of skincare a little easier!

First of all, you need to determine what your skincare concerns are. Do you want to fight acne, hyperpigmentation, ageing, dryness or excess oil? Do you have dry, oily, combination or normal skin? Once you have decided what your main concerns and skin type are, you can more easily determine which products will work for you.

You also need to have a think about your budget. Skincare products vary in price hugely, so it's worth having an idea of what you'd like to spend before starting to look for a new product or regime.

Once you have an idea of what you *might* like to try, I would recommend doing a good amount of research into specific products before you buy them. Look online at blogs and video reviews or ask shop assistants what they think of individual products in comparison to what you're currently using. This will help to avoid wasting money on dud products. If you can speak to an expert in the area, even better! Every time I get the chance to speak to a professional facialist or skincare expert, I always pick their brains on the best product for my skin type!

THE BASICS

I think a lot of the confusion surrounding the world of skincare comes from people not really understanding what each product does or when and how to use it. Here's my guide to the skincare basics.

Makeup Remover

A lot of people don't realise that makeup removers aren't necessarily cleansers. A lot of them are formulated to simply remove makeup, not to thoroughly cleanse the skin. Experts recommend using a makeup remover, then a cleanser, or to wash your face twice using the same cleanser to remove all residue from the skin. It is for this reason that I firstly use a makeup remover or micellar water (Bioderma's Sensibio H_2O is widely renowned as the best on the market), then a cleanser when I'm wearing makeup.

Cleanser

There are so many different varieties of cleanser. Whether you go for a milk, gel, balm, oil or cream depends on your skin type, preference and individual skin concerns. My personal favourites are balm formulas, as they are very effective at removing any last scraps of makeup and dirt, yet they don't leave your skin feeling stripped or tight. They are also great if you have dry or sensitive skin.

Toner

A toner is a liquid that delivers beneficial ingredients directly onto the skin after cleansing. Depending on the formulation, they can also 'close' the pores and smoothe the texture of the skin, ready for the application of moisturiser and makeup. It is applied on a cotton pad, or sprayed directly onto the skin after cleansing. This is a step that a lot of women skip, but using a toner (in my opinion at least) is one of the most pleasurable steps in a full skincare routine, as it makes your skin feel smooth, soft and clear. Toners containing alcohol are common, but somewhat controversial in the skincare world, as alcohol can be drying and can cause irritation. I personally love using Caudalie's Eau de Beauté spray as a toner, and to refresh my skin throughout the day.

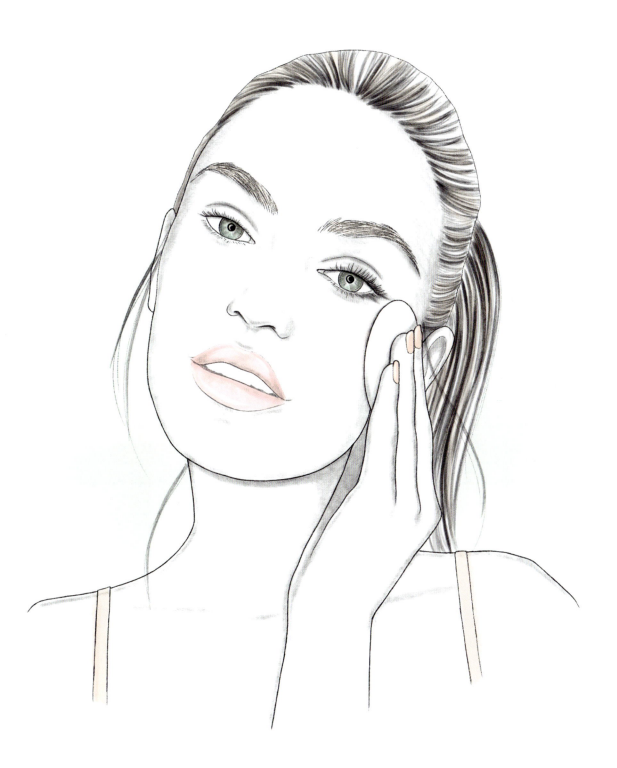

Serum

Serums are one of the skincare items I get asked about the most. A lot of women don't really understand what they are meant to do, or when you are meant to use them. Serums are a targeted treatment specifically formulated for certain skincare concerns. They contain a higher concentration of active ingredients than moisturiser and should be used before moisturising, both in the morning and evening. Face oils tend to fit into the serum category too. Although they are different to the traditional serum formulation, they are used in place of serum, at the same point in your routine. I only use a serum or oil when my skin needs a little extra boost of hydration, usually when I'm travelling or in the winter.

Moisturiser

Moisturiser is a cream product that is formulated to hydrate the skin. It may also offer other benefits, such as anti-ageing, oil control or anti-pigmentation, based on the individual formulation of the product. There is often a misunderstanding when it comes to the idea of 'hydration' vs 'oil'. Oily skin can still be dehydrated and therefore those with oily skin should still moisturise. The right formulation of moisturiser can actually help to balance oily skin. My personal favourite is from The Organic Pharmacy.

Eye Cream

Although eye cream is often associated with more mature skin and anti-ageing products, women should start using eye cream from their early twenties if they want to prevent the first signs of ageing, as the eyes are usually where wrinkles first start to appear. Choosing an eye cream that is right for your age and skin type is essential. A lot of them are very heavy, thick formulas, which are often inappropriate for younger skin. You should apply your eye cream as the very last step in your skincare routine. Use your ring finger to gently tap the product onto your skin, along your orbital bone. You should be applying the product right up to the outer corner of your eyes (where you would develop 'crow's feet') and even up onto the brow bone if you want to. Don't simply apply it underneath your eye, as it can easily migrate into your eye and cause irritation. Also be sure to avoid applying your regular moisturiser in this area, as it is much more delicate than the rest of your face. Your regular face cream (especially if it is anti-ageing or anti-acne) may irritate the area. I use a brightening eye cream from First Aid Beauty called Triple Duty. It's amazing for moisturising, de-puffing and banishing dark circles in one step.

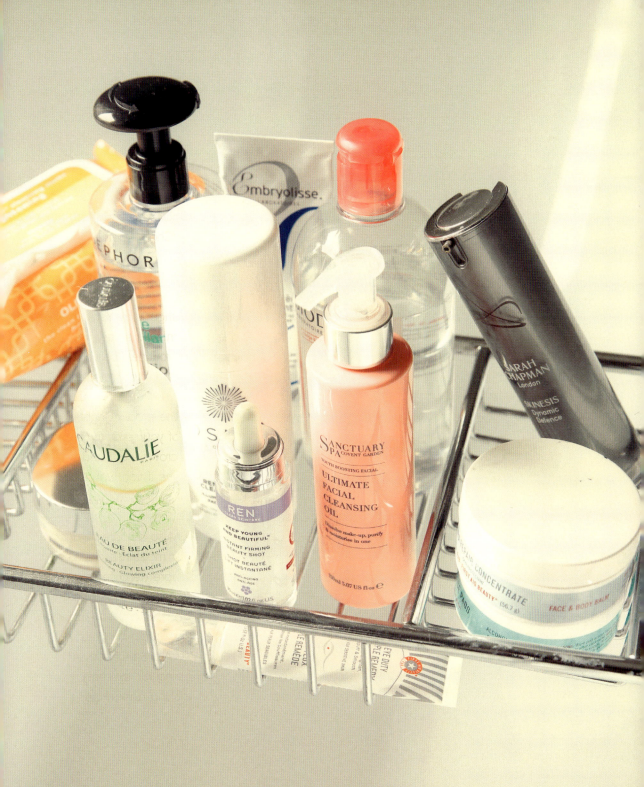

DIY Face Masks

You don't have to spend a fortune to get clear, glowing skin! There are a lot of natural ingredients you can find in your local supermarket that work wonders in a DIY face mask. Mix your own mask based on your individual skin problems using my ingredient guide below.

Tip: It's always best to start with a thicker base (avocado, banana, cooked oats or mango) and add in the dry or liquid ingredients, so you get a good consistency that is easy to apply.

Avocado

Avocados are jam-packed with nutrients, proteins and vitamins. They are a great ingredient for hydrating all skin types, are also good for anti-ageing and can help reduce dark spots. They also have amazing reparative properties that can help soothe sunburn and leave your skin baby-soft. Mash or blend them thoroughly before putting them in your mask.

Egg Whites

Whipped egg whites make a great addition to your DIY face mask if you're looking to minimise pores and temporarily lift and tighten the skin. They also contain protein, which encourages tissue repair and growth.

Oats

Putting oats into your face mask has many benefits. They are a great, gentle exfoliant and can therefore make your treatment a two-in-one mask and scrub. They are also a great solution for oily skin and are gentle enough not to strip or dry out the skin at the same time. They provide relief from itchy, irritated skin, so are good for those with sensitive skin. Use cooked oats, unless you only want them for exfoliation purposes. Cook them as you would to eat for breakfast, then let them cool to room temperature before mixing with your other ingredients.

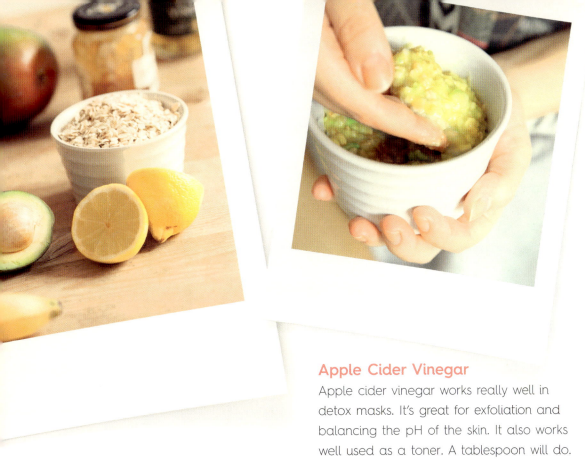

Apple Cider Vinegar

Apple cider vinegar works really well in detox masks. It's great for exfoliation and balancing the pH of the skin. It also works well used as a toner. A tablespoon will do.

Banana

Rich in potassium and antioxidants, bananas are good for moisturising the skin, and also for oil control and acne. They are known as 'nature's botox' and are a good, natural anti-ageing ingredient. Mash them well before adding them to your recipe.

Mango

Packed with vitamins A and C and beta-carotene, mangoes are amazing for brightening your skin and reducing dark spots. Mash the mango flesh well before adding it to your mask.

Honey

Naturally anti-bacterial and packed with antioxidants, honey is great for acne-prone skin. Manuka honey is even better, as it has stronger anti-bacterial properties. Honey is also great for adding moisture and clearing out the pores.

Lemon

The natural acids in lemon juice can help exfoliate your skin and will brighten your complexion, reduce dark spots and even your skin tone. Squeeze lemon juice into your mask for an added boost. It also works very well with honey for an acne-fighting treatment.

Five Minute Makeup

It's pretty rare that we ever have as much time as we would like to get ready in the morning. If you're really in a rush, here's how I streamline my beauty routine to ensure I look put-together even when I only have a few minutes to spare.

Cleanse and moisturise. If your skin is in good condition, you need less makeup. It only takes a few minutes to properly cleanse and moisturise your skin, so never skip this step, no matter how much of a hurry you're in!

Skip foundation. Just use concealer to cover up any problem areas. This way you can still even your skin tone and hide any major imperfections, but save a lot of time.

Use a small pencil brush and some **dark eye shadow** to line your eyes. This is much quicker than using eyeliner, as you don't have to be too precise, and it instantly gives your eyes definition and makes your lashes look fuller.

Curl your lashes. Curling your lashes instantly makes your eyes look bigger and more awake, and it only takes about ten seconds!

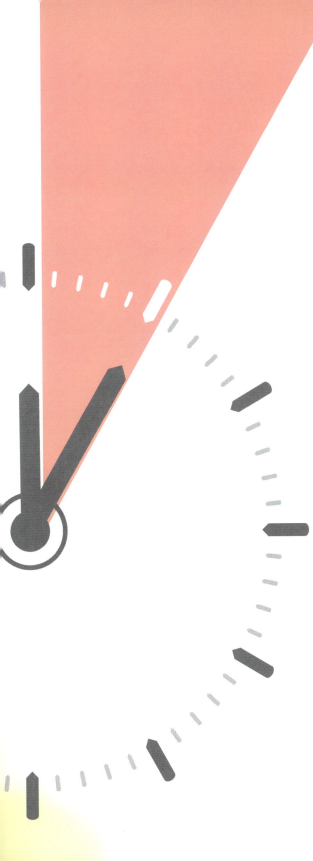

Don't pass on mascara! If there's one makeup item I can't live without, it's mascara. It can make you look so much more awake and put-together and only takes a minute to apply. Pick one with a big, bushy brush for the quickest application.

If you're in a hurry, **use products that are multi-use,** as it will shave down the time it takes to get ready! My favourites are lip and cheek creams you can use as a blusher and lipstick.

Go for a plait or side-pony. Both of these options take under two minutes to style, but look more polished than a simple ponytail or messy bun. They also work really well if you don't have time to wash your hair. Dry shampoo is also a great option if you are time-limited, as it freshens up your roots and adds volume and texture at the same time, which works really well when plaiting your hair.

Plan ahead! If you know you're going to be in a rush in the morning, plan your makeup and outfit the night before, so that you can easily streamline your routine.

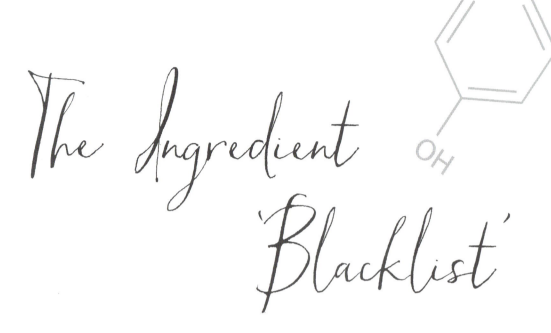

The Ingredient 'Blacklist'

Over the past few years there have been a number of ingredients that have become quite taboo in the beauty world. Although many of them still appear in approved, safe-to-use products, they have a bad reputation. So what do they really do and should you be using them?

PARABENS

Perhaps the most debated cosmetic ingredient, parabens are chemical preservatives commonly used in cosmetics and toiletries. Some research has found parabens in cancerous breast tumours, but as yet there is no direct link between products containing parabens and cancer. They also mimic the effect of oestrogen in the body, and have therefore become a controversial ingredient in many respects. They are becoming easier to avoid, as many brands and products are now

'paraben free' as a result of increasing concern about their effects on the female body. Contrary research concludes that parabens are metabolised before they enter the blood stream, and therefore cannot be harmful, so it's hard to know what to think. My personal stance is to try to avoid them if the product is staying on my skin (face cream, serum or body lotion) but I'm not too worried if it is washed off (shower gel, shampoo) and doesn't get left on the skin to absorb.

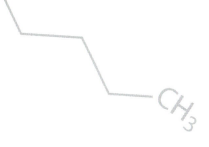

MINERAL OIL

Mineral oil is a cheap by-product of making petroleum. It's a clear, odourless oil that is widely used in moisturising creams and cosmetics. Although it isn't closely linked to anything sinister, it acts as a barrier on the skin and can lead to clogged pores and breakouts in some people. It also gets criticised (especially when used in expensive skincare products) for not having any specific benefit for the skin and being a cheap alternative to using natural plant oils. Others argue that because it acts as a barrier, it helps to keep moisture in your skin. It is the main ingredient in many basic moisturising creams recommended by doctors, including aqueous cream. My stance on mineral oil is in the middle. I don't go out of my way to avoid it, and I don't mind it being used in cleansing products, as it can be effective at removing makeup, but when it comes to expensive creams and lotions, I wouldn't splash the cash for mineral oil-based products.

SILICONE

Silicones are a group of synthetic ingredients used in cosmetics which can be easily identified on a list of ingredients, as they usually end in '-cone' or '-conol'. They are derived from sand and started to become popular for use in cosmetics in the 1950s. They have many different uses in cosmetics, including waterproofing, retaining water, smoothing the hair and skin, and protecting the hair shaft. Silicones used in hair products have long been a subject for debate in the beauty world. They 'coat' the hair, so while leaving it looking shiny, smooth and healthy at first, after prolonged use, they can weigh the hair down, making it look limp and lifeless. Having quite thick, unruly hair myself, I actually quite like using silicone-based products. I just make sure I use a clarifying shampoo regularly to avoid them building up in my hair (my favourite is from Unite). There are also concerns that silicones build up in the environment, with many environmental groups discouraging their use out of concern for aquatic environmental damage.

PHTHALATES

These chemicals are used in cosmetics to help hold scent or colour, and are therefore often found in nail polishes and perfumes. They are hard to spot on lists of ingredients, as they are often part of the simple 'fragrance' label, but they may also be listed as DBP (dibutyl phthalate) or DEP (diethyl pthalate). These chemicals can disrupt your endocrine system by mimicking hormones and this has been linked to a variety of different health problems. They have different results depending on which hormone is mimicked, but in the case of oestrogen, they have been linked to breast cancer, weight gain and infertility.

FORMALDEHYDE

Formaldehyde-releasing chemicals are used as preservatives or hardeners in many cosmetics. These chemicals release a very small amount of formaldehyde over time into the formula, helping to preserve the product. This is a concern, as formaldehyde is a known carcinogen (it causes cancer), though there are strict limitations as to the amounts of these chemicals companies can use in cosmetics. They are most commonly used as a hardener in nail treatments. Formaldehyde-free formulas are fairly easy to find (although often a little more expensive), so if you're concerned, go for a brand like Butter London or Essie. You can find more extensive lists of formaldehyde-free brands online.

SULPHATES

Sulphates are chemicals commonly used in shampoos, body washes and cleansers. They are essentially foaming agents. Sulphates are controversial for a few different reasons. Firstly, they have been linked to skin irritation and dry skin. They have also been blamed for releasing carcinogenic by-products (although the levels of these are very, very low and not expected to have a significant effect) and they also provide an environmental concern for many, as they are synthetically produced from a non-renewable source. Sulphates are worth avoiding if you have issues with sensitive or dry skin, but otherwise they are one of the lower-level concerns on our blacklist.

TOLUENE

Toluene is a solvent used in nail polishes. It helps to break down other components in the formula to ensure a smooth, easy application. It is controversial because long-term exposure to very high doses has been proven to cause cancer and reproductive problems. There has been a lot of debate about the use of toluene in nail polishes, and whether or not it is harmful in the small quantities found in them, and therefore many brands have stopped using it.

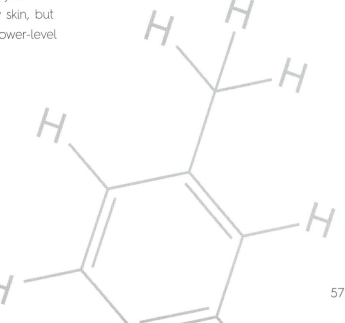

10 Quick Tips

Do Your Research

The internet is an incredible resource for makeup reviews. Look up at least three different reviews of a product before you buy it. This will help to save you money in the long run as you'll be much less likely to waste your money on bad products.

Fix a Smashed Eye Shadow

Add a few drops of rubbing alcohol to the broken powder. If there are still big chunks of product, break these up with the end of a clean knife first. Add your alcohol, then cover a coin with a clean cotton cloth and re-press the product down into its compact or pan. This will save you from having to throw it away, or making a huge mess in your makeup bag!

Makeup Expiry Dates

A lot of products have a little 'open lid' symbol on them, with a number of months. This tells you how long you can expect them to stay fresh for after opening. For mascara and liquid liner, it's best to throw them away after three months of use, but other products last longer. Foundations can keep for up to a year. Lipsticks and powder products up to two years if you take good care of them. Store your makeup in a cool, dark, dry space (avoid keeping makeup in your bathroom as the steam makes it a breeding ground for bacteria). Look out for any change in consistency, smell or colour. This tells you it's time to throw it away!

Rosehip Oil for Scars

If you have a fresh cut or burn that you think will scar, apply a drop of rosehip oil every morning and night. Massage it over the area to help reduce the chance of getting a scar. Rosehip oil is also a great natural, affordable, multi-use product to have in your bathroom cabinet as it's also a wonderful oil to use on your skin at night to prevent ageing. You can also use it to moisturise your hair and nails!

Get Longer Lashes

Apply castor oil to your lashes at night to encourage growth. Use a clean mascara wand to coat them from root to tip before you go to sleep. This will help keep them moisturised and in great condition, preventing breakage, thinning and helping them to grow. Remember that eyelashes have an average lifespan of just 150 days before they shed and re-grow, so make this a regular step in your beauty routine to see long-term effects.

Make Any Lipstick Matte

If you don't wear matte lipstick all the time, don't waste your money buying a matte finish. Instead, apply a little bit of translucent powder to your lips and then blot with a little bit of tissue. This will give any glossy lipstick a beautiful matte finish.

Make Your Eyes Look Bigger

Line your lower waterline with a nude coloured eyeliner. A lot of people recommend using white, but nude or flesh-toned liner looks a lot more natural. Most people won't even realise what you've done, but your eyes will look noticeably larger. To further enhance the look, use a little bit of matte eye shadow (either dark brown or black) and smudge it lightly, just underneath your lower lash line.

Make Plucking Painless

Try plucking your eyebrows after you shower. This will open up your pores, making it less painful to pull out the hairs. This also applies for waxing or epilating your body as well.

Store Your Liquid Liner Upside-Down

This will ensure you get a nice, solid black line every time and also prevent it from drying out as quickly.

Melt Your Makeup!

If you like to apply your foundation and concealer with your fingers, hold it between your fingertips for 10 seconds before applying it to your skin. This will warm the product and make it blend in to your skin even more easily.

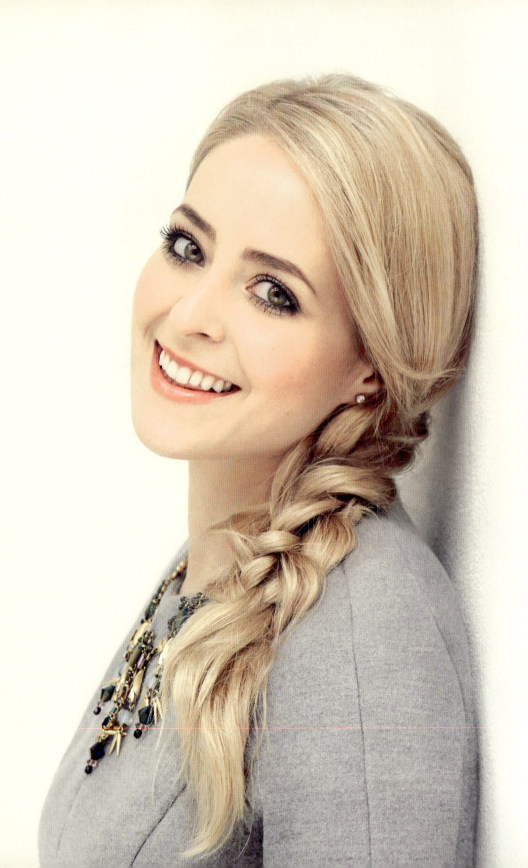

Hair

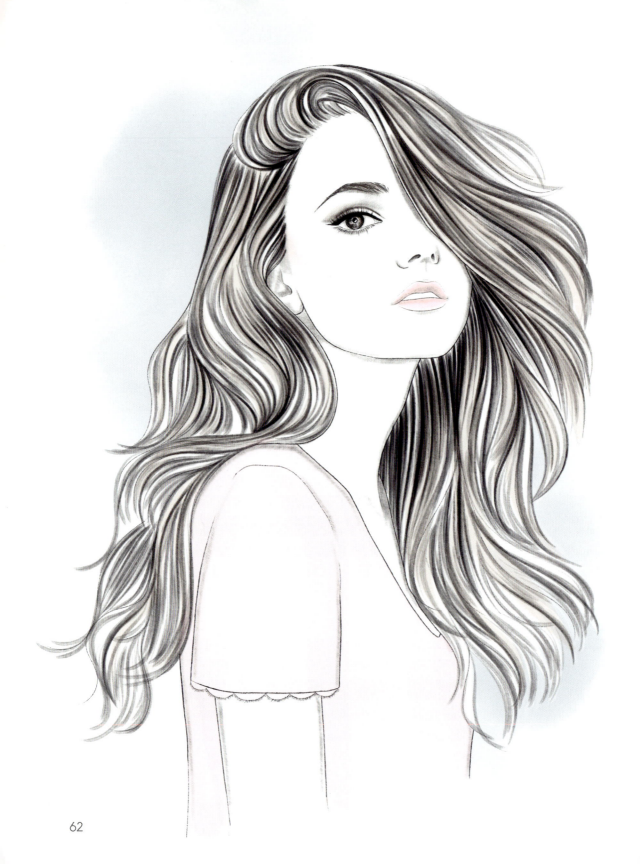

Introduction

The idea of a 'bad hair day' affecting you emotionally seems silly, superficial and, quite frankly, over the top, but your hair really can have a huge impact on your confidence and self-esteem, whether you consider it trivial or not. Having good hair has the ability to change your outlook on the day from the get-go. No matter the length, style or colour of your hair, everyone likes to keep it in the best condition possible and looking its very best. This chapter is packed with my tips for looking after your hair, no matter what you put it through, as well as quick and easy hairstyles to ensure you never have a bad hair day again.

5 Easy Hairstyles for Every Day

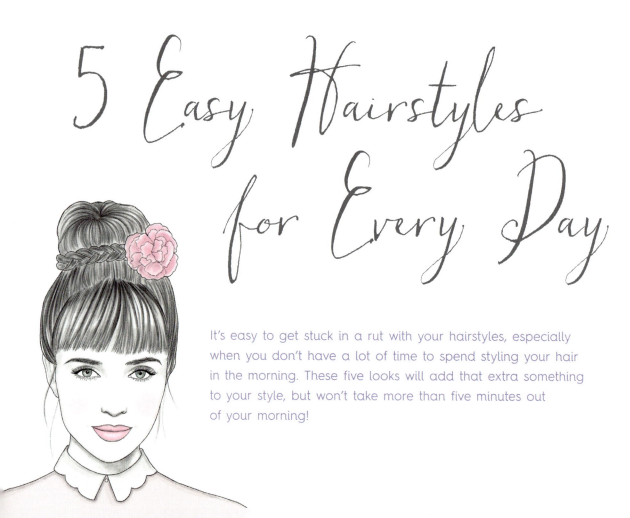

It's easy to get stuck in a rut with your hairstyles, especially when you don't have a lot of time to spend styling your hair in the morning. These five looks will add that extra something to your style, but won't take more than five minutes out of your morning!

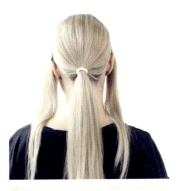

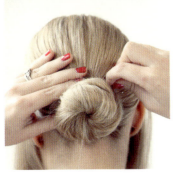

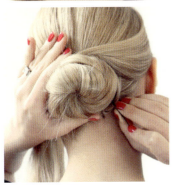

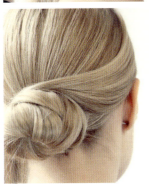

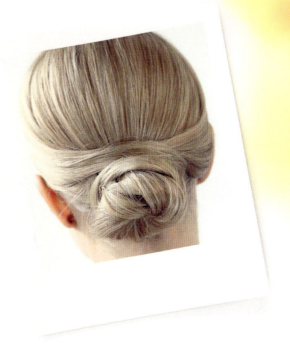

THE CRISS-CROSS BUN

Add a little fun to your everyday bun by leaving two strands out at the front. Tie up your bun at the nape of your neck, as you would normally do, then take one of the loose strands at a time and wrap it around the far side of the bun, so that they 'criss-cross'. Pin the strands into place underneath the bun, so it looks neat and tidy.

THE TUCK AND COVER

This is a great way to wear headbands without having to spend a lot of time arranging them in your hair. It's also a good way of covering up the plain band at the back of your head. Put your headband on over the crown of your head, leaving the band at the back exposed. Working from your ear to the nape of your neck, take inch-wide sections, twist them so they are smooth, then tuck them over and under the back of the headband. Add more hair to the section and keep tucking until you reach the centre. Repeat this process on the other side and you'll be left with a simple but chic-looking up-do. Use a little hairspray to lock it into place. You might also need a bobby pin at the centre point to secure the final section into place.

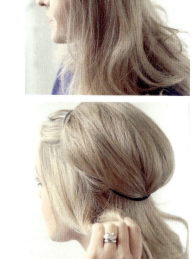

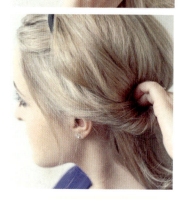

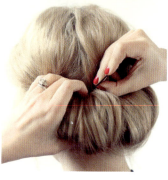

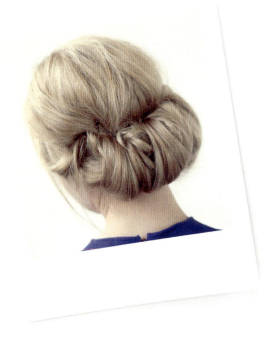

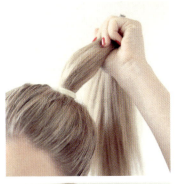

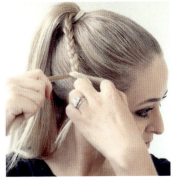

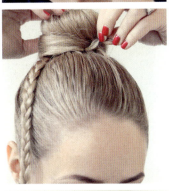

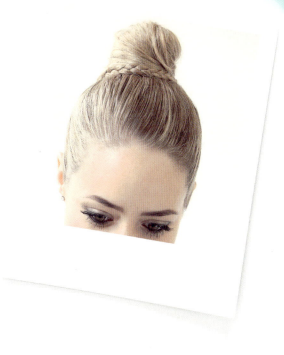

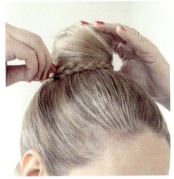

THE BRAID AND BUN

Tie your hair into a ponytail on top of your head. Take out a small section at the side and plait it. Twist the remaining hair into a neat bun and pin it into place. Then run the plait around the base of the bun and pin it into place with a bobby pin.

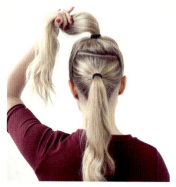

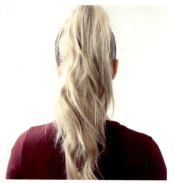

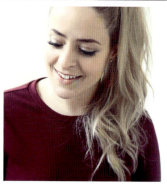

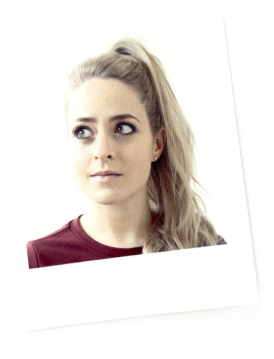

THE SUPER-LONG PONY

This neat little trick makes your ponytail look twice as long without the need for extensions. Divide your hair horizontally into two sections, and tie each into a ponytail: one at the top of your head, tied as a high pony, and the other just above the nape of your neck. Position the top pony so that it covers the one below. This will give the illusion of super-long 'mermaid' hair! Add a few waves to the ends of your hair for added texture.

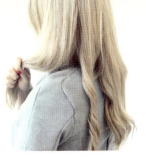

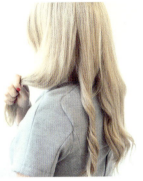

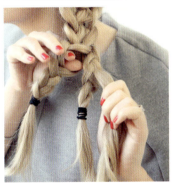

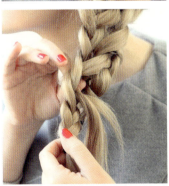

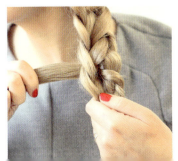

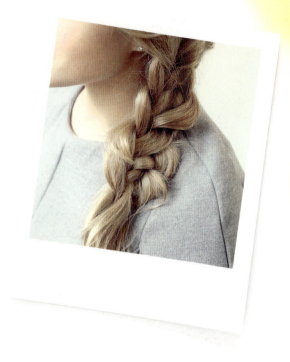

THE TRIPLE BRAID

This takes a few minutes longer than the others, but it's guaranteed to attract compliments and it's really simple to do once you get the hang of it. Pull your hair over to one side of your neck and divide it into three sections: two big sections, with a smaller one in the middle. Braid the two larger sections and secure them with a hair tie at the end. Then take the tiny section and hook it through the centre of each larger braid, alternating between the two braids. This effectively ties the two larger braids together and leaves you with an extra-wide 'mermaid' braid. When you've finished, secure the end with a small elastic hair-tie and gently pull out the braids to loosen it and make it look messy.

DIY Hair Masks

As with face masks, many ingredients you'll find in your fridge have amazing benefits for your hair. I still use packaged hair masks, but making your own can be a fun way to switch up your routine, and can also give your hair a serious boost without the added chemical nasties. DIY masks are also a great option if you have specific hair or scalp concerns, as you can tailor them to suit your needs. Here are my three favourite recipes for targeted DIY hair masks that will help you tackle your hair woes.

Tip: For short hair, halve the amount of everything to avoid waste.

THE MOISTURE MASK

If you have dry, damaged hair, DIY hair masks are definitely for you! There are so many deeply moisturising ingredients that are probably already in your kitchen cupboard. My favourite recipe is one of the simplest, and it's based on super-nourishing coconut oil. You can buy cosmetic-grade coconut oil very cheaply at your local pharmacy or drugstore. It's solid at room temperature, so when mixing it with other ingredients, warm it up first, either in your hands or on a low heat on your kitchen stove. Honey is also a natural humectant, meaning it attracts and retains moisture, so it's great for locking moisture into your hair. Bananas are packed with vitamins and natural oils that can help lock moisture into the hair shaft and are also a great addition if you have a dry or sensitive scalp.

Ingredients

2 tablespoons of coconut oil
1 tablespoon of honey
1 banana (very ripe)

Instructions

Soften the coconut oil with your hands or melt it on the stove. Then pop all of the ingredients into a blender and blend until smooth. Massage the mixture into the lengths and ends of your hair while it's dry and leave it for 20–30 minutes before shampooing as normal. I would recommend shampooing twice to remove any oil residue.

Results

You'll be left with super-soft, smooth locks. It's also great for taming frizz!

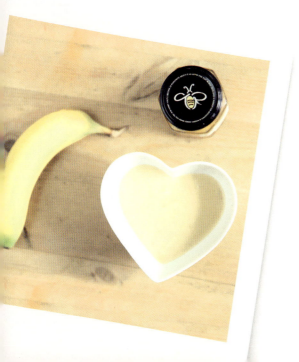

THE SHINE AND GROWTH SOAK

If your locks are looking dull and lifeless, try this easy DIY mask to add shine, remove product build-up and leave your hair looking smooth and silky. It's also great for those who are trying to grow their hair, as it contains lots of good growth-promoting ingredients. Avocado is packed with vitamins A, D, E and B6, which can encourage hair growth and deeply moisturise your hair. Olive oil is also a wonderful ingredient for promoting growth, as it contains antioxidants, and it has been used as a natural hair conditioner for centuries. Egg yolks are full of protein that strengthen and repair your hair, adding moisture and shine. Finally, apple cider vinegar helps to restore the optimal pH balance of the hair and removes any product build-up that can restrict hair growth.

Ingredients

½ an avocado (as ripe as possible)
2 tablespoons of olive oil
1 egg yolk
1 tablespoon of apple cider vinegar

Instructions

Mash the avocado with a fork until smooth, then add the other ingredients and mix thoroughly. Massage into dry hair and leave for 20 minutes before shampooing as normal.

Results

Your hair will feel soft and nourished but less weighed down, and it will have a beautiful shine.

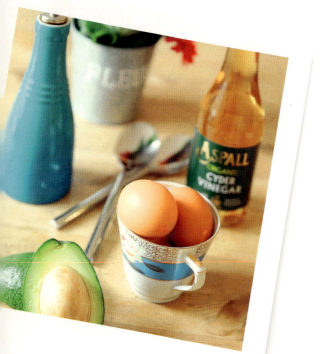

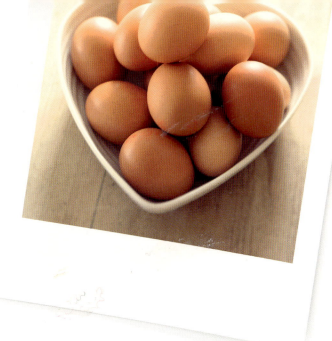

THE OIL-CONTROL TREATMENT

If you have oily hair, try out this quick treatment that will help soak up any excess oil and remove build-up at the same time. Egg whites contain enzymes which help to absorb the natural oil from your scalp and hair. Lemon juice is a natural astringent, so helps to reduce oil production from the pores on your scalp, and apple cider vinegar helps to balance the pH of your scalp and remove any residue on your scalp and hair shafts.

Ingredients
3 egg whites
2 tablespoons of apple cider vinegar
1 lemon

Instructions
Whisk the egg whites until smooth and frothy. Add the vinegar and whisk until blended. Add the juice from the lemon and mix together. Apply it to your scalp and roots of your hair and leave for 5–10 minutes. It's best to do this in the shower, as the mixture is very runny and can be messy to apply!

Results
You hair will feel super-clean, volumised, shiny and will stay oil-free for longer.

Colouring Your Hair

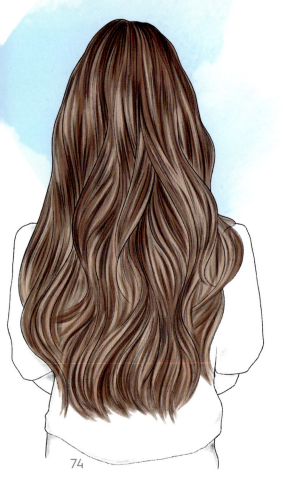

Whether you're colouring for the very first time or just fancy a change from your usual shade, dyeing your hair can be a great way to transform your look or enhance your natural assets, but it can also be a minefield. Here are my top tips to help make the colouring process an easy one, from choosing the right shade for you, to actually achieving the colour you have in mind, to minimising the damage to your hair and making your new colour last as long as possible.

CHOOSING A COLOUR

Look at your hair, skin, eyes and eyebrows to determine your natural tones and try to stick within the same family. If you have warm, yellow tones in your skin and hair, going for a cool-toned hair colour may look odd. Keeping your hair colour in sync with your skin tone is often the key to finding the most flattering, natural-looking colour for you.

BE REALISTIC

If you're going for a big change, don't expect to get the perfect result the first time. Especially if you're going from dark to light, it can take months to achieve the colour you want. It's also a good idea to take your time and change your colour gradually, in order to minimise the damage to your hair.

PREP YOUR HAIR

Use an intensive moisturising mask a couple of days before colouring, as moisture will help the hair to hold pigment better. Don't wash your hair the day you colour it, as the natural oil on your scalp will help protect it from the chemicals in the dye, especially if you have a sensitive, irritable scalp.

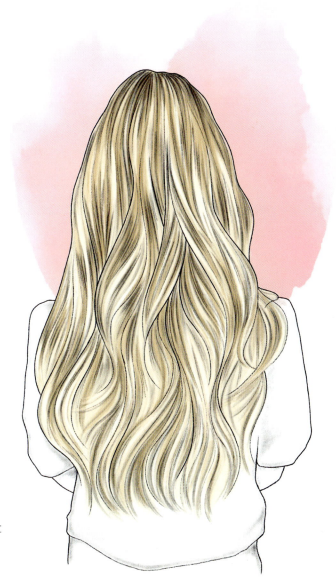

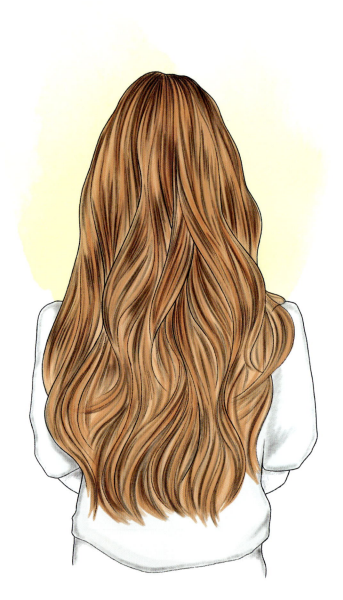

DON'T FORGET TO DO A SKIN TEST FIRST

Most salons insist on doing a skin test at least 48 hours before you have your hair coloured with them for the first time, but it's also important to do this if you're dyeing your hair at home, in case you have a reaction to the chemicals in the dye. Apply a very small amount of the dye behind your ear at least 24 hours before you colour your hair. Check the area the next day for any redness or irritation.

DON'T BE SHY

If you get your colour professionally done, don't be afraid to tell your stylist exactly what you want and ask them any questions you may have throughout the process. Taking in a photo of what you want is also a great idea, as another person's idea of a colour might not be the same as yours, but remember that you have to be realistic with what is achievable. You're not always going to be able to replicate someone else's hair exactly.

DYEING AT HOME

If you choose to dye your hair at home, don't go for a huge change the first time you try it. Don't forget to put Vaseline along your hairline and on your ears, to prevent your skin from staining. Always buy a semi-permanent dye if you're not 100 per cent sure about the colour or application process. Experts also recommend going for one shade lighter than you want, as colours (especially reds) usually come out a little darker than they look on the box.

INVEST IN SPECIALIST PRODUCTS

If you've gone to the effort and expense of colouring your hair, use products that will help to maintain it. Clarifying or dandruff-treatment shampoos often strip the colour out of the hair, so they are best avoided on fresh colour. Choose something that is not only formulated for coloured hair, but also for your specific choice of colour and tone. This will minimise the maintenance needed to keep your colour looking fresh. Wella make a great selection of shampoos and conditioners formulated for different shades of coloured hair, and I also personally love Unite's range for blonde hair.

COUNTERACT THE DAMAGE

Colouring your hair is damaging, especially if you're lightening it with bleach. Counteract the damage by using intensive treatments at least once a week, to keep your hair in good condition. Check out my recipes for DIY hair masks for cheaper and more natural alternatives to expensive conditioning treatments.

KEEP AWAY FROM CHLORINE AND SUNSHINE

Chlorine not only damages hair but also affects the pigments in it (both natural and artificial), so it's best to avoid chlorine as much as you can. Tie your hair up or wear a swimming cap in the pool. UV rays are also very damaging to the hair, so if you're out in the sunshine, it's best to wear a hat or use products with UV protection to help maintain the quality and colour of your hair.

Growing Your Hair

Some of the questions I get asked most frequently are how I grew my hair so long, and how I keep it in good condition while still colouring it frequently. Whilst it is true that growing your hair simply takes *time*, there are also some other factors that affect your ability to grow your hair long.

KEEP SPLIT ENDS IN CHECK

The most important thing to do when you want to grow your hair is to keep an eye on any damage to the ends. Breakage is the main reason your hair doesn't appear to be growing. It's a total myth that *cutting* your hair makes it grow faster. You should trim your hair regularly when you're trying to grow it, but only to limit split ends and damage from spreading up the hair shaft and causing breakage. Keep a close eye on the condition of your ends and get a trim when you notice they are damaged. For some this may be every six weeks, for others, up to three months.

AVOID DAMAGE FROM WASHING

In order to minimise damage, limit washing your hair to two or three times per week, as washing it too often strips the natural oils and can leave it brittle and more susceptible to damage. Massage your scalp when you wash it. This will help to stimulate your hair follicles and encourage growth. Also, take the time to rinse your hair in cool water after you've washed it. This not only leaves you with shiny locks, but helps to smooth the shafts of the hair too, which can help to reduce breakage. Brushing your hair also helps to stimulate your hair follicles, so aim to brush your hair (and scalp) for two minutes, twice a day. Remember to only brush your hair when it's dry if you can, as your hair is more susceptible to breakage when it's wet.

REDUCE DAMAGE FROM STYLING

Heat styling is often the main source of damage and breakage, and therefore limits hair growth. For most of us, it's simply unavoidable, but try letting your hair dry naturally if you want to curl it afterwards, or blow-dry it straight with a brush to avoid the need for straighteners. Also, don't forget to use a heat-protection spray or lotion whenever your hair comes into contact with heat. Try to avoid strong chemicals or dyes. Bleach is very drying and damaging to the hair, but also try to avoid perms or any other strong chemical treatments if you want to grow your hair.

HEALTHY HAIR FROM THE INSIDE OUT

What you put inside your body really does affect the quality of your hair and the speed at which it grows. If you eat a healthy, well-balanced diet, your hair will not only grow faster, but will be in better condition. Some of the best foods for hair growth include salmon, walnuts, oysters, sweet potatoes, eggs, spinach, lentils, Greek yoghurt, blueberries and chicken.

Taking a good multi-vitamin supplement is also beneficial for encouraging hair growth. You can choose one specially formulated for your hair and nails, but simply making sure you're getting all of your essential vitamins will make a difference.

STAY HYDRATED!

Drinking plenty of water is recommended as a solution for almost every beauty concern, as it really does improve most aspects of your body. Drinking lots of water not only helps to keep your hair hydrated, but it also helps to flush out toxins and therefore your hair will be stronger, not as dry and less susceptible to breakage.

Tip: To help condition your hair and encourage growth at the same time, try making your own protein-rich hair mask with eggs (see pages 70-73 on DIY hair masks for my favourite recipes).

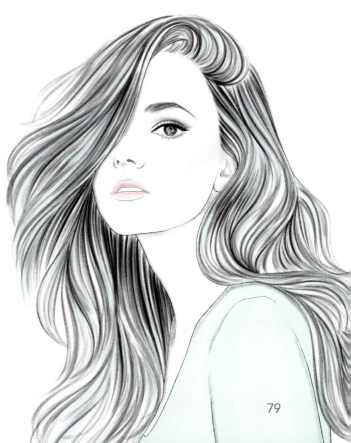

10 Quick Tips

Use a Silk Pillow Case

Because silk is much smoother than cotton, using a silk pillowcase reduces the friction between your hair and your pillow. This will help to minimise damage, but it will also mean you wake up with smoother, less knotty hair in the morning.

Squeeze Your Hair Dry

Rubbing your hair dry with a towel can ruffle the cuticles and cause damage and tangles. Gently squeeze your hair with your towel to remove excess water.

Go for a Medium Heat Setting

Don't automatically set your heat-styling tools to the hottest setting, as it may be hotter than you need. The optimal temperature for maximum styling potential with minimal damage is around 180°C (350°F), although it does depend on the type and condition of your hair. Using hair tools on a very low heat setting can also be damaging, as you're more likely to repeat the process numerous times to achieve the results you're looking for.

Use an Overnight Treatment

Overnight masks are becoming more popular, and are less messy than you might think! There are lots available in the shops, but I simply like to massage coconut oil into the ends of my hair, tie it in a tight bun and leave it overnight. When I wake up and wash it out, my hair is super-soft and shiny!

Stop the Slip!

Spray your kirby grips or bobby pins with dry shampoo or hairspray before you use them. This will stop them from slipping out or moving in your hair. A lot of people also don't realise that they are designed to be used with the bumpy side *against* your scalp for optimum hold.

Backcomb with a Toothbrush!

If you like the effect of backcombing, but have fine hair which is easily damaged, try using a soft-bristled toothbrush instead of a comb. This will help to minimise damage. You can also use it to keep flyaways at bay by spraying the bristles with a little hairspray and gently smoothing any stray hairs down.

Get Serious Volume at Home

Spritz in a volumising spray at the roots, then flip your hair over and rough-dry it upside-down until your hair is 90 per cent dry. Flip it back over and finish drying with a big, round brush for an at-home blow-dry with serious volume.

Set Your Hair Style

Just as heat can change your style, cold can help set it. Give your hair a gentle blast of cold air when you've finished heat-styling, to help it stay in place all day.

The Gym Pony

When tying your hair up in the gym, stack three hair ties in a row, to keep your hair off the back of your neck and free from sweat.

The Four-Minute Rinse

One of the main causes of dull hair is not rinsing products out thoroughly. It takes about four minutes to fully rinse shampoo out of long hair, so make sure you take your time in the shower to keep your locks shiny.

Fashion

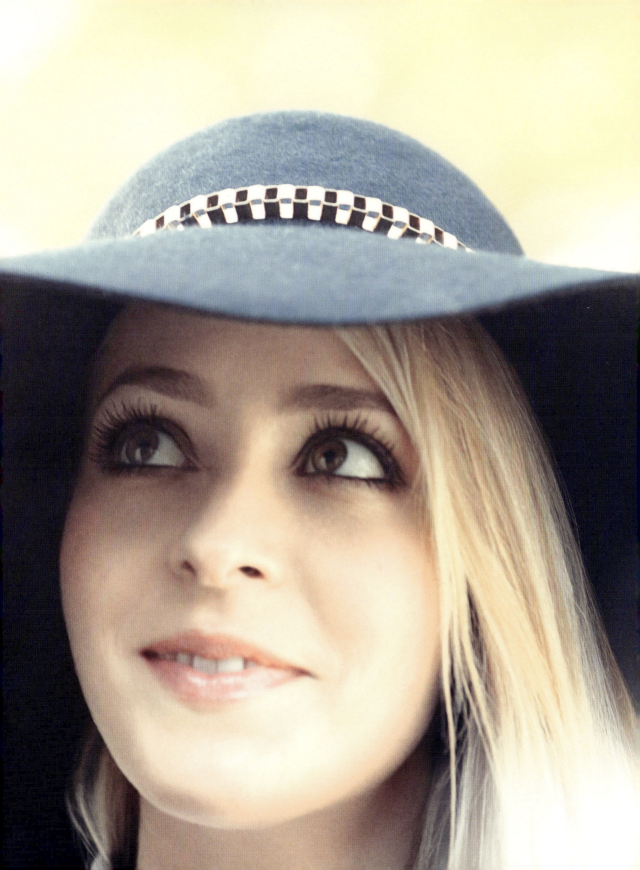

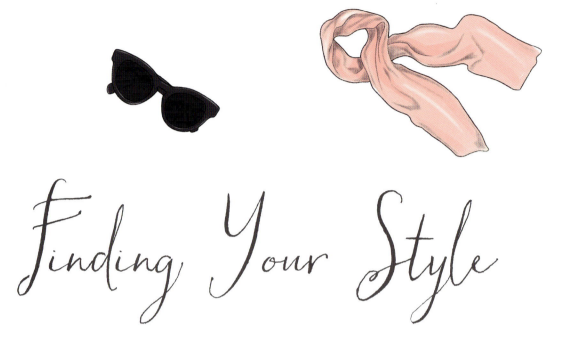

Finding Your Style

Putting a finger on what exactly your style is can be tricky. Sometimes it's easy to sway in between styles and never really work out what suits you best. Here is my advice for helping you to discover your individual style so you can feel comfortable and confident at the same time.

DRESS FOR YOURSELF

Wear the outfits that *you* feel most comfortable in. The moment you start dressing for someone else, you lose some of your own personal style.

DON'T BUY SOMETHING BECAUSE YOUR FRIENDS LIKE IT

I've done this a few times and learnt the hard way. If you're shopping with friends and they just *love* something that you try on, but you're not sure, don't be persuaded to buy it. The same goes for clothes you see someone else wearing – if you know deep down that they won't go with anything else in your wardrobe, steer clear!

MAKE SURE IT FITS

Clothes that fit you *really* well look instantly more stylish than ill-fitting ones. If it doesn't fit, *don't* buy it! (Unless of course you can get it adjusted.)

DON'T CARE WHAT PEOPLE THINK

Easier said than done! If you do care a little too much and feel self-conscious in an outfit or item of clothing, maybe it's not for you.

PAY ATTENTION TO THE SMALL DETAILS

Even the tiniest of details can define your style: the jewellery that you never take off, or that perfect shade of lipstick that pulls your look together. Small touches like these become your style trademarks, so try to incorporate them into your look as a whole.

ONLY FOLLOW TRENDS THAT SUIT YOU

There are some trends you know are just never going to fit in with your style or suit your figure, no matter how fabulous they look on others. My own no-go trends are creepers and crop-tops. They look fantastic on some, but will never look good on me, so I know not to go there.

PUT YOUR BEST FOOT FORWARD

Never wear shoes you can't walk in! Tottering around in high heels never looks stylish.

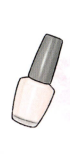

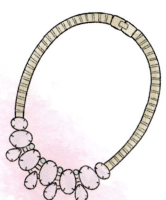

Shortcuts to Looking Stylish

We've all been there. You go to an event thinking your outfit is great, only to arrive and be left thinking that every other girl in the room looks so much more stylish than you. Here are five easy steps to being one of those girls . . .

CONFIDENCE

Fifty per cent of being stylish is being confident in your choice of outfit, and confidence is something you *can* fake. It's all about posture, poise and eye contact. If you've chosen a bit of an outlandish outfit, make sure you hold your head high and walk like you feel totally confident wearing it.

GET SOME STYLE INSPIRATION

If you ever feel like you're stuck in a style rut and find it hard to follow trends, find a celebrity or blogger who you like the style of and take inspiration from their outfits. Sometimes trends are hard to pull off, but you never know until you try them yourself. There are so many trends I've hated until I've worn them myself, then fallen totally in love with them. (Hello, playsuits and wedge trainers!)

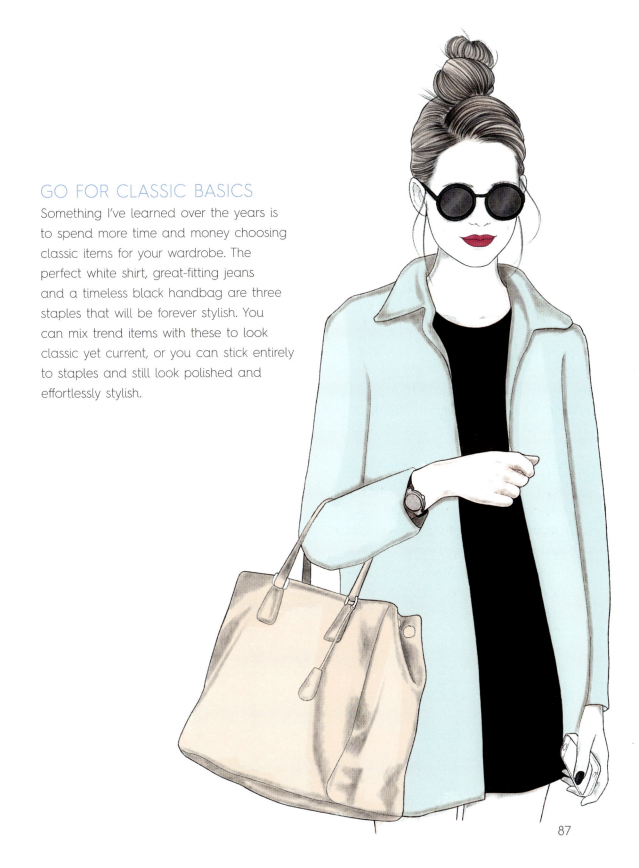

GO FOR CLASSIC BASICS

Something I've learned over the years is to spend more time and money choosing classic items for your wardrobe. The perfect white shirt, great-fitting jeans and a timeless black handbag are three staples that will be forever stylish. You can mix trend items with these to look classic yet current, or you can stick entirely to staples and still look polished and effortlessly stylish.

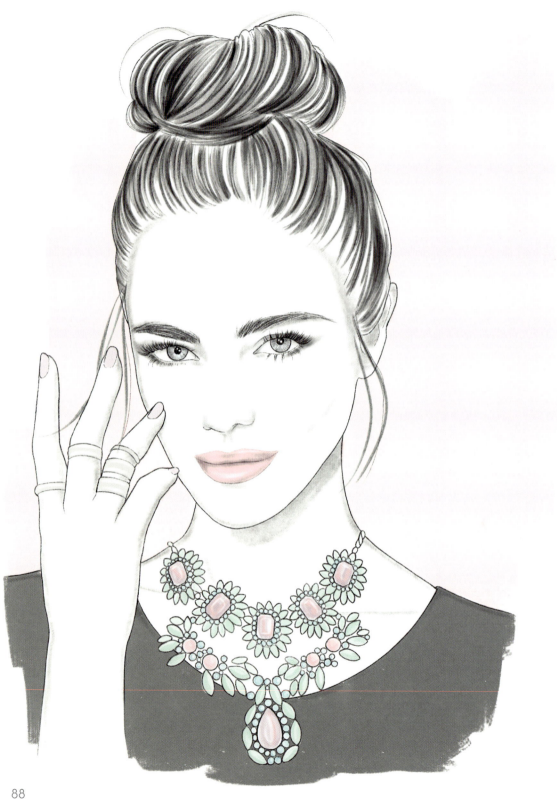

'All of the most stylish girls I know are always a little messy looking.'

WEAR A DARING ACCESSORY

Pairing classic pieces with a daring accessory like a hat or statement bag can make an outfit. Hats can feel quite intimidating to wear, but something about them is inherently stylish. They feel super glamorous and are an easy way to take your outfit up a notch in the style stakes. Whatever accessory is hot that season, buy an affordable version first and wear it a few times. I do this with new accessory trends I'm not 100 per cent sure about, and more often than not, I end up buying more than one after giving the affordable version a go.

DON'T LOOK TOO 'PUT-TOGETHER'

All the most stylish girls I know are always a little messy looking. You don't want to look like you've put too much thought into your look, as that can often seem like you're trying too hard. This doesn't mean you have to be scruffy all the time, just add a little imperfection to your look. Try adding a little messy texture to your hair, slightly mismatching accessories, or a lip stain instead of a lipstick.

Wardrobe Essentials

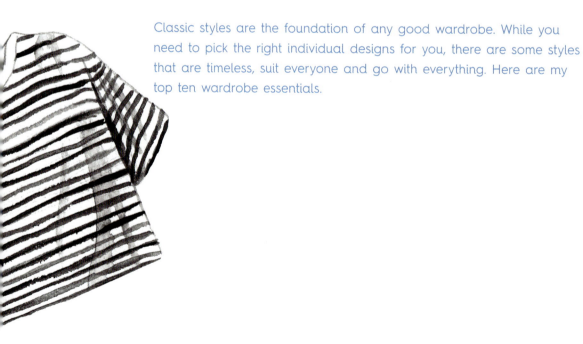

Classic styles are the foundation of any good wardrobe. While you need to pick the right individual designs for you, there are some styles that are timeless, suit everyone and go with everything. Here are my top ten wardrobe essentials.

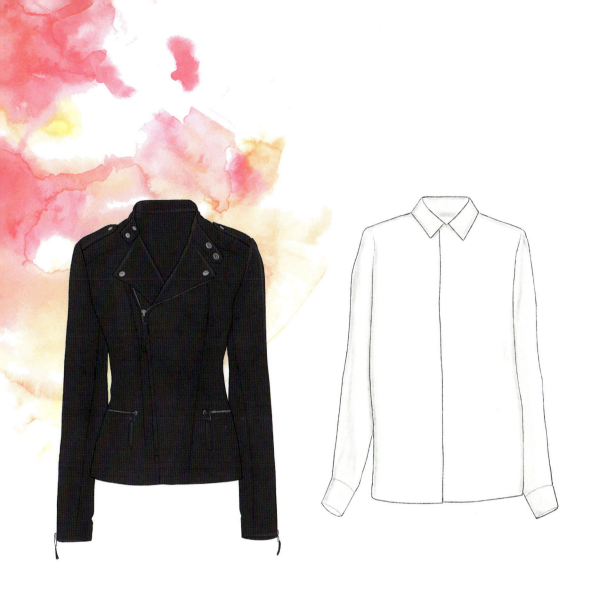

BLACK JACKET

Whether it's a black leather biker jacket or a classic blazer depends on your personal style, but a lightweight black jacket is my number one wardrobe essential. It's the perfect way to cover up, smarten up a scruffy outfit or dress down a cocktail dress.

WHITE SHIRT

Finding the perfect white shirt can be hard, but once you've found it, you won't be able to live without it. Dressed up or down, a crisp, white, perfectly fitting shirt has timeless class.

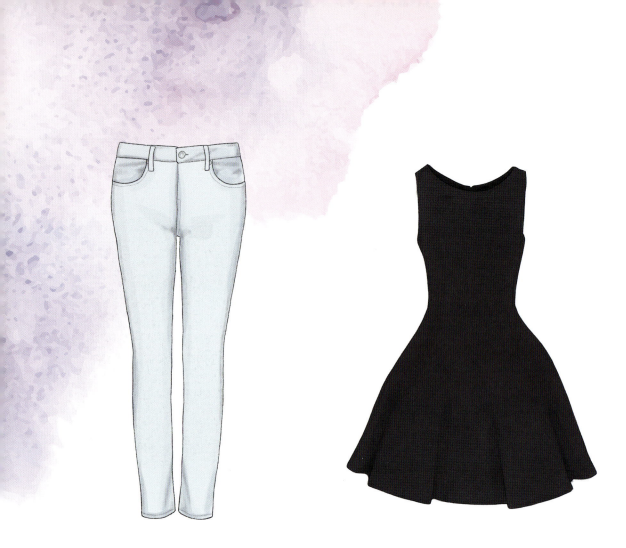

GREAT-FITTING JEANS

If you haven't found your perfect pair of jeans yet, check out my guide on pages 96–99. Whether they're black, indigo or acid wash, ripped, faded or pristine, finding your perfect jeans is the key to pulling off countless casual looks.

LITTLE BLACK DRESS

The typical girl probably has a couple of LBDs in their wardrobe, but finding one that suits your figure perfectly can see you through pretty much any occasion. Pair it with statement accessories to make it look different every time. There are now a few websites solely dedicated to little black dresses, with advice on which styles will suit which body shape – www.littleblackdress.co.uk is one of the best.

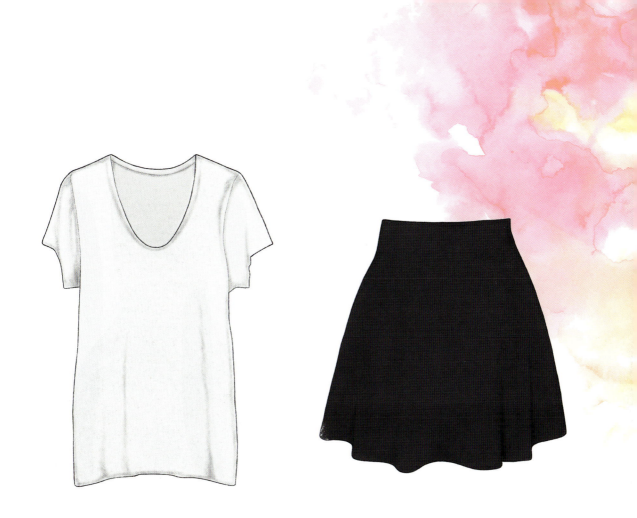

BASIC WHITE OR GREY T-SHIRT

Another casual staple. Once you find the perfect style for you, buy a few in a couple of different colours, as you never know when you'll find the perfect fit again.

BLACK SKIRT

Different styles suit different body shapes, but a classic black skirt can be part of endless different outfit combinations. I usually end up re-dyeing my staple black skirts every year or so, as they often fade after numerous washes. (The same goes for black jeans: you can easily get them looking fresh and jet-black again with at-home dye.)

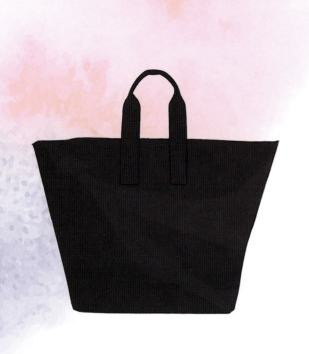

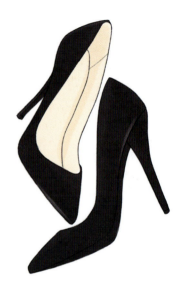

BLACK HANDBAG

While statement bags might catch your eye in the shops, a classic black bag is the most versatile accessory there is. Choose a medium-sized one you can dress up or down and use in the daytime or evening. Detachable or chain straps are preferable for increased versatility.

BLACK HIGH HEELS

I wear my black pumps at least ten times as much as any of my other heels. A patent finish will last longer than suede or natural leather, but any plain black pump will go with every outfit. They can easily dress up jeans and a T-shirt, or pair them with a statement dress to keep it looking chic and not over-done.

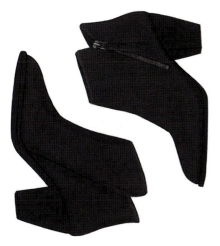

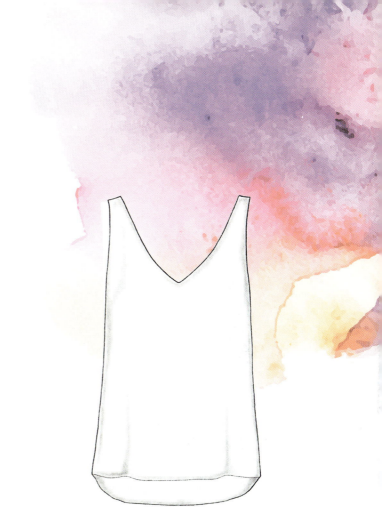

BLACK BOOTS

Whether you're into ankle boots, biker boots or riding boots, a good quality black boot will see you through many winters. I get mine re-soled and heeled every year in preparation for the colder months. If you do this before they get totally worn down they can (and will) last you for years, as you'll avoid damaging the heel.

TANK TOPS

Even if you never wear them alone, basic strappy tops are a total wardrobe essential. I always have a couple in black, white and grey. Whether you wear them under sheer tops or layer them up in the autumn and winter to keep warm, no wardrobe is complete without them!

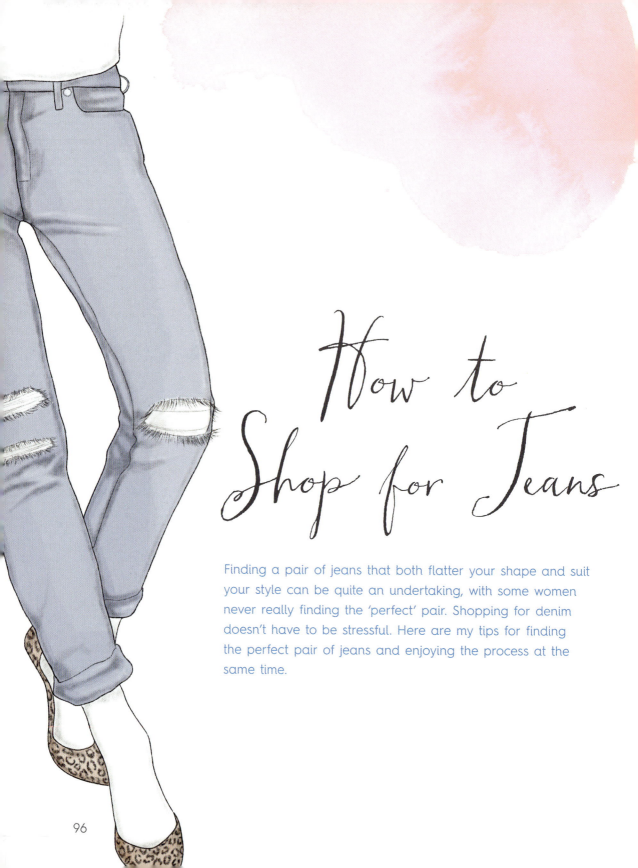

How to Shop for Jeans

Finding a pair of jeans that both flatter your shape and suit your style can be quite an undertaking, with some women never really finding the 'perfect' pair. Shopping for denim doesn't have to be stressful. Here are my tips for finding the perfect pair of jeans and enjoying the process at the same time.

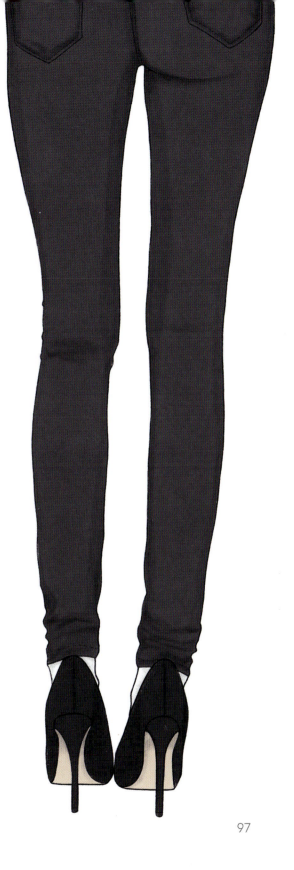

TAKE YOUR TIME

When you're looking for a new (perfect!) pair, make sure you have an hour or two set aside to try on a variety of different cuts to find which suits you best. Also be sure to try a variety of different brands. If you're in the denim department of a larger store, often the sales assistants really know their stuff, so ask for their advice on the best choices for your body shape, which brands might suit you and which are the most comfortable.

STICK TO THE RIGHT CUT FOR YOUR BODY SHAPE

Boyfriend jeans are best suited for boyish figures. If you're curvy, choose a cut with a slight flare or a straight leg, to balance out your hips and bum. If you're petite, go for a slim-fit style, cropped at ankle length, which will make you look taller.

TAKE A COUPLE OF DIFFERENT TOPS AND SHOES WITH YOU

Take along a selection of tops and shoes which you think you might want to wear with your new jeans. This will make sure you're confident you can wear your jeans with a variety of different outfits.

IF YOU FEEL SELF-CONSCIOUS, OPT FOR DARK DENIM

Dark or black denim is always more flattering than lighter shades. They are also more versatile, as you can dress them up or down.

PERSONALISE YOUR PAIR

If they aren't the perfect length, get them professionally taken up. If you like distressed jeans, but the perfectly fitting style don't come ripped, do it yourself! There are loads of tutorials online showing you how to do this. Whatever you decide to do, make sure you wash your new jeans twice before adjusting them, as denim tends to shrink a little on the first and second washes.

TAKING CARE OF YOUR FAVOURITE JEANS

The rule about not washing your jeans for six months after buying them is not only gross, but it's also not true for most jeans, as they have usually already been pre-washed, distressed or faded, so the denim has already been worn into shape. To help preserve the shape and colour of your jeans, wash them inside out on a cool wash (with the fly and button done up) and let them air-dry naturally. You can also throw half a mug of vinegar in with your denim wash to stop darker jeans from fading as quickly.

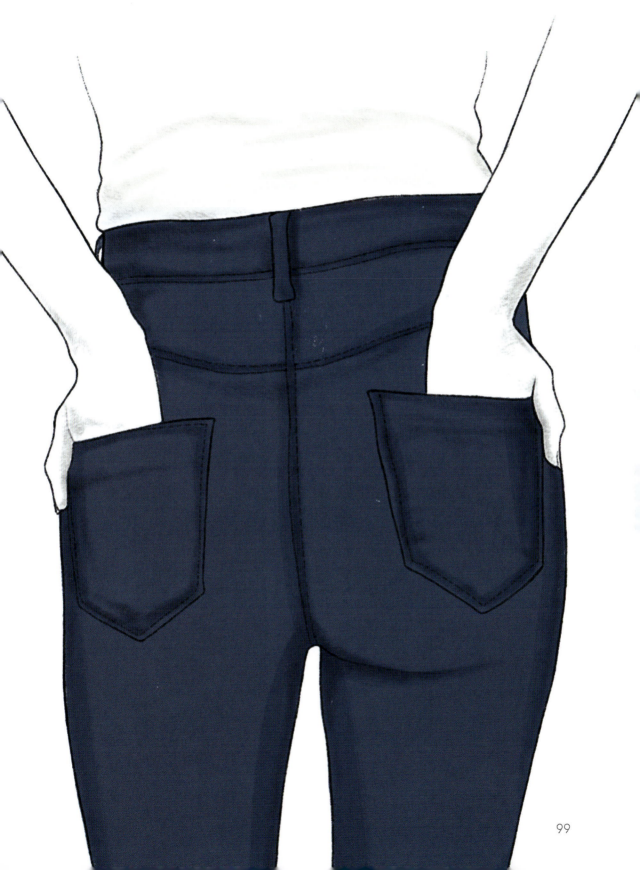

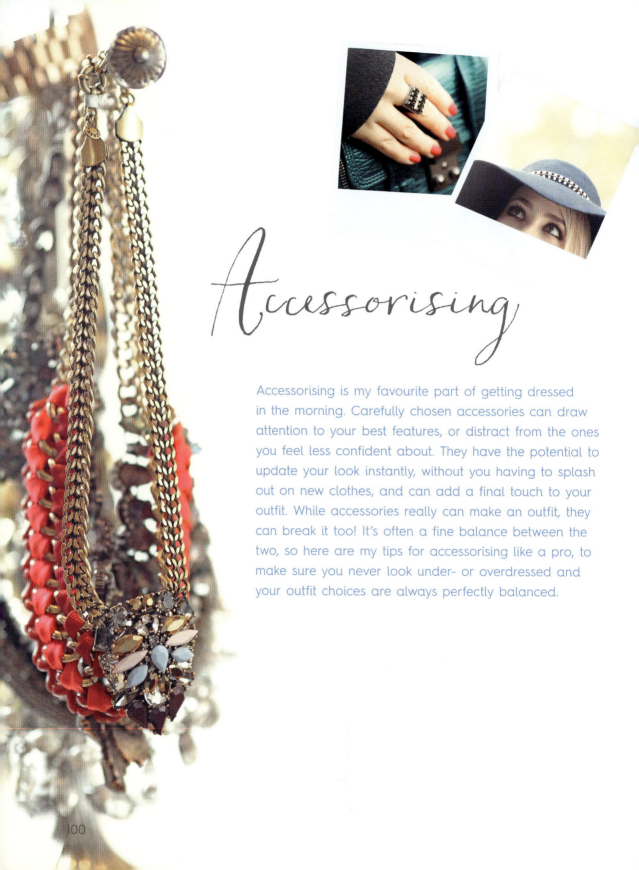

Accessorising

Accessorising is my favourite part of getting dressed in the morning. Carefully chosen accessories can draw attention to your best features, or distract from the ones you feel less confident about. They have the potential to update your look instantly, without you having to splash out on new clothes, and can add a final touch to your outfit. While accessories really can make an outfit, they can break it too! It's often a fine balance between the two, so here are my tips for accessorising like a pro, to make sure you never look under- or overdressed and your outfit choices are always perfectly balanced.

THINK ABOUT YOUR WHOLE OUTFIT, NOT INDIVIDUAL PIECES

I find laying my outfit out on my bed before putting it on is an easy way to ensure everything works together without having to try everything on. Be wary of pairing busy clothing with busy accessories, as this can make your whole outfit look a mess. If you've chosen to wear a graphic print or pattern, keep your accessories simple, so you don't overcomplicate your look.

YOU DON'T HAVE TO MATCH YOUR ACCESSORIES

The days of matching your handbag to your shoes are long gone, but do try to keep them coordinated. Your whole look should work in harmony. You don't want colours, textures or shapes fighting with each other for attention. I always try my best to match my metals, although not necessarily when it comes to jewellery (mixing metals looks gorgeous when they are stacked). Think about the hardware on your handbag and your shoes, for example. Grey boots with silver hardware will fight with a brown bag with gold hardware. There are no strict rules, but make sure your choices work together harmoniously.

EACH PIECE SHOULD ADD SOMETHING TO YOUR OUTFIT

Take a minute to think about how what you're putting on will make a difference to your overall look. If an accessory isn't doing something positive for your outfit, replace it with something else. Keep this in mind when you're shopping for accessories and try to choose things that flatter your shape, size and skin tone. Oversized bags may look great on tall girls, but can swamp the petite amongst us. Similarly, dainty rings will make your fingers appear longer and slimmer, while chunky rings can often make them look shorter and wider, so try before you buy!

SPACE OUT YOUR STATEMENT PIECES

It usually works to stick to one statement accessory at a time, as you don't want to look like your accessories are fighting for attention. If you do want to wear a couple of different statement pieces together, make sure they are well spaced out. For example, a statement necklace paired with chandelier earrings will look unbalanced and is very hard to pull off, but statement shoes and a necklace paired together can look great.

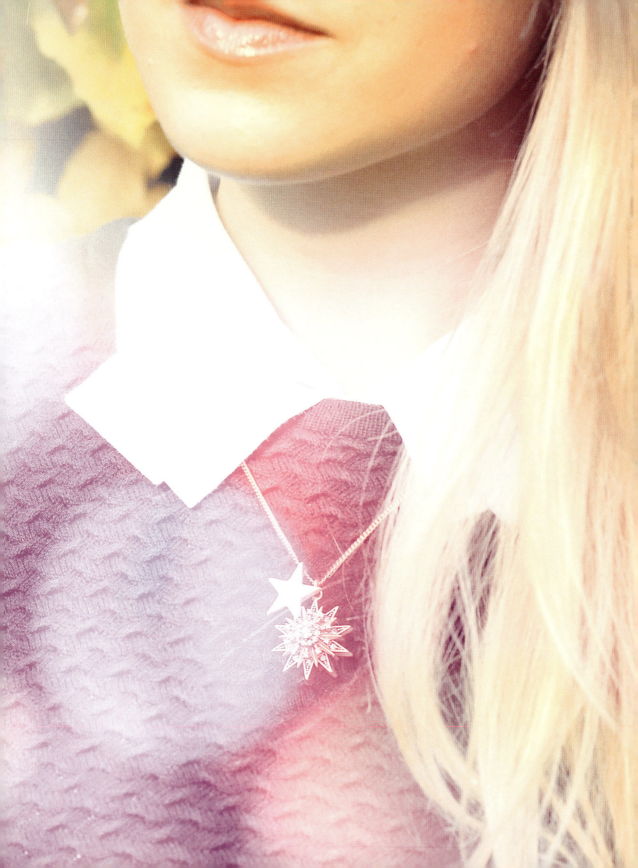

ACCESSORISE ACCORDING TO THE OCCASION

Over-accessorising or wearing accessories that impede what you're doing that day is never a good look. Think struggling to type because your fingers are laden with chunky rings, overheating under your perfectly layered scarf when out shopping, or juggling with a clutch bag and grocery bags. Accessories are fabulous, but be realistic about what you choose to wear and where you choose to wear it!

DON'T BE SCARED TO GO BOLD!

Fun-coloured accessories are easier to pull off than bright clothing, so they are a great way to wear bold colours if you don't feel confident wearing them elsewhere. They are also an easy way to update your look with a colour-of-the-moment, enabling you to add something on-trend to many different outfits.

DON'T OVER-ACCESSORISE OR UNDER-ACCESSORISE

As the great Coco Chanel famously recommended, 'Before you leave the house, take a look in the mirror and take one thing off.' While this is great advice for those who tend to over-accessorise, if you tend to under-accessorise, you may need to add an accessory before you leave! A better way to think about it is to take a good look at your outfit, including your coat and handbag, before you leave the house, then decide if you need to add or subtract anything.

Tip: If you buy a cheap ring as an instant style update, coat the inside with clear nail polish to stop it turning your finger green!

Trends vs. Investments

Typical advice when it comes to investment shopping is to not follow trends and invest in classic designs. Realistically, you aren't always drawn to the classic, neutral staples you know you should be saving up for. So how can you balance the temptation to splash all of your savings on that utterly fabulous of-the-moment designer handbag with the age-old advice telling you to go for the classic, quality number?

IT'S ALL ABOUT BALANCE

Yes, classics will see you through the years, but you also have to think about adding a little personality to your wardrobe. As the late Oscar de la Renta said, 'Fashion is about dressing according to what's fashionable. Style is about being yourself.' Some trends last longer than others, so investing in a more 'trendy' designer piece that really suits you and your style can be an investment if you choose the right design. Try choosing a trendy design in a neutral colour, or a classic design in a statement colour. You're essentially going halves. If you really love something, then it fits your natural style, which is more important than what's in fashion at that moment.

CHOOSE PRACTICAL MATERIALS

No matter which style you choose to invest in, beware of delicate fabrics, exotic leathers and very light colours. No matter how good the quality, delicate items age more quickly and are likely to wear out after less use, regardless of design. For handbags, textured leather ages the best, as it is particularly durable. A handbag in saffiano, faux-crocodile or caviar-textured leather will last you much longer than one made of finer, smooth leather. For shoes, it is best to steer clear of light colours, satin and suede if you want them to last a long time.

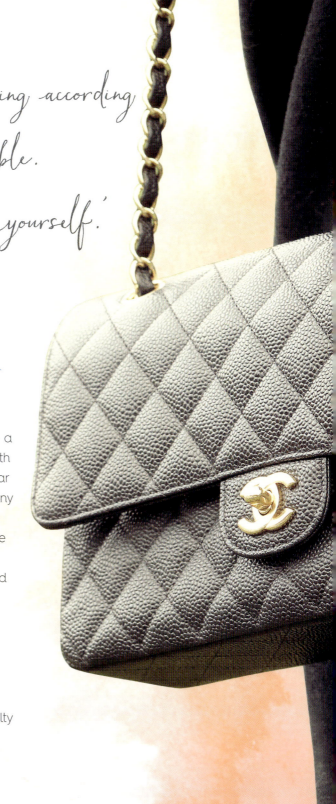

'Fashion is about dressing according to what's fashionable. Style is about being yourself.'

OSCAR DE LA RENTA

GOOD-QUALITY BASICS AREN'T ALWAYS EXPENSIVE

You don't always have to invest in basics; simply choose them wisely. Some basics, like a classic coat or black handbag, are well worth spending a little more on, but items that wear out or stain easily, like white T-shirts and skinny jeans, are better off coming from a more affordable brand (my favourite basic tees are from H&M, and I love Zara's skinny jeans). Affordable doesn't always have to mean bad quality, you just have to look harder to find great-quality items on the high street.

AVOID IMPULSE BUYS

Always give yourself some time to think big purchases over. If you're going to invest in your wardrobe, make sure you don't feel guilty or regretful afterwards.

How to Make High Street Look High End

You don't always have to spend a lot to achieve an expensive look. There is definitely an art to making high-street items look expensive. Here are my top tips.

IT'S ALL IN THE MIX

Above anything else, designer accessories have the ability to make any outfit look more expensive. I think handbags do this the best, as they are statement items that are often instantly recognisable as being designer. You can also wear them with virtually any outfit (which you can't do with clothing items), so one high-end item can make your whole wardrobe look more expensive. If handbags aren't your thing, coats are also a great way to do this in the winter, as you generally wear the same coat with lots of different outfits.

GO FOR INSPIRED, NOT FAKE

If you don't have the budget or desire to invest in designer pieces, buying designer-inspired items will get you the look for less. Although it's often tempting to buy a knock-off version of that handbag you've been lusting after for years, most fakes are pretty obvious to anyone who's seen the real thing, and *you'll* always know it's a fake, so you'll never value it as highly as the real thing, and you'll still want the legit version (trust me, I've been there). Try looking for styles that are instead *inspired* by designer items. Zara are particularly great at recreating a certain style so that it looks different from the real deal but has the same effect on your overall outfit.

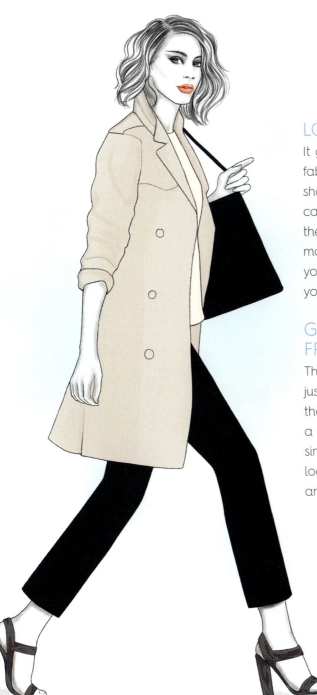

LOOK FOR QUALITY AND CUT

It goes without saying that better-quality fabrics look more expensive. This is where shopping online is often difficult, as you can't touch the items before you buy them. Clothing that fits well also looks more expensive. If high-street items don't fit you like a glove, get them adjusted to fit you perfectly.

GET INSPIRATION FROM FRENCH FASHION

There's something about Parisian style that just *looks* expensive. Stunning simplicity is the Parisian signature style, but if you take a closer look, it's more about keeping it simple than spending thousands. Get the look for less by opting for muted tones and plain designs.

KEEP IT CLEAN

Obviously it's always a good idea to keep your clothes clean, but it's also worth taking a little time to make them look immaculate too. Perfectly laundered clothing always looks more expensive, so taking good care of your clothes is an easy step towards a more beautiful wardrobe.

KEEP YOUR MAKEUP AND HAIR POLISHED

'Polished' doesn't necessarily mean 'a lot'. A full face of makeup can sometimes look 'cheaper' than a simple, clean look. Concentrate on giving yourself a glowing, flawless complexion, with groomed brows and bright eyes. When it comes to hair, nothing looks better than a fresh blow-dry. If you can learn to blow-dry your own hair to a near-professional level at home, this is an easy way to make any outfit look more beautiful.

IF ALL ELSE FAILS, WEAR BIG SUNGLASSES

Sunglasses have an air of glamour about them – the bigger the better! A great pair of sunnies have the ability to give you a confidence boost and make you look more sophisticated in an instant.

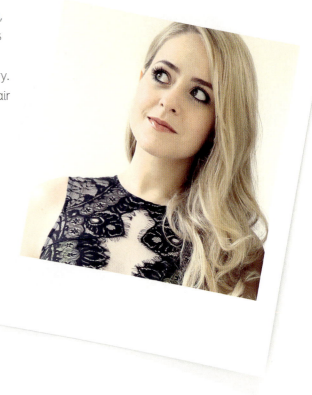

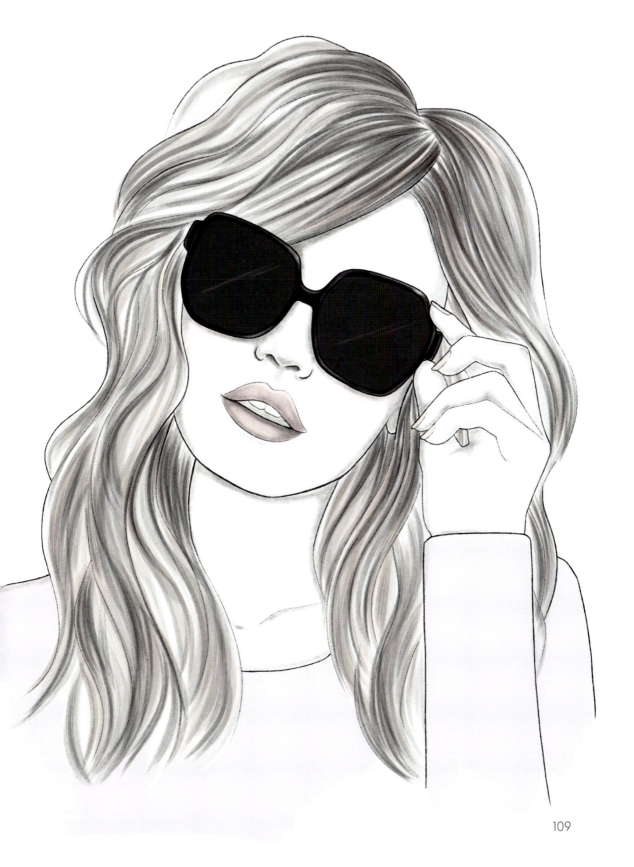

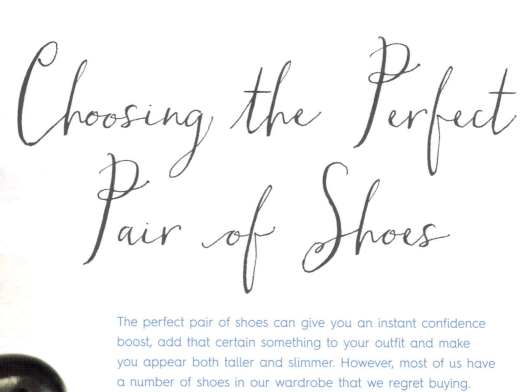

Choosing the Perfect Pair of Shoes

The perfect pair of shoes can give you an instant confidence boost, add that certain something to your outfit and make you appear both taller and slimmer. However, most of us have a number of shoes in our wardrobe that we regret buying. Whether it's because they're uncomfortable, hard to walk in or difficult to style, we've all wasted our money on the wrong pair of shoes. Here are my tips for finding the perfect pair, every time.

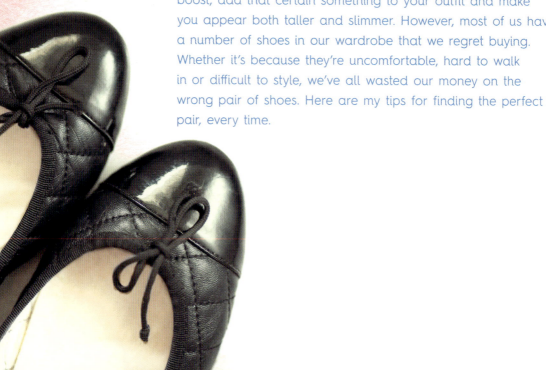

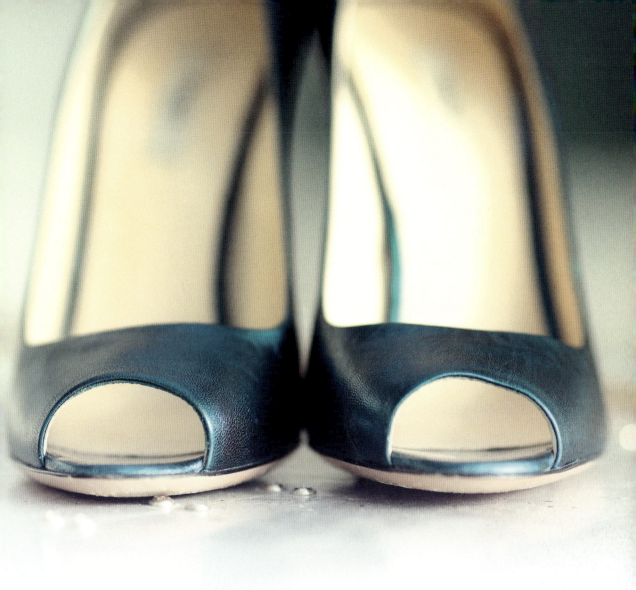

CHOOSE A NATURAL MATERIAL THAT BREATHES

This will allow your feet to breathe, make them cooler and more comfortable to wear and therefore reduce the chance of them becoming smelly! If they have ventilation holes or a specially designed heel that provides ventilation, even better.

GET THE RIGHT SIZE

Sizes can vary from shop to shop, so if your normal size is a little too big or small, ask to try on half a size up or down. Sometimes it may not be the design of the shoe that is causing the problem, it might be the brand in general runs bigger or smaller than average.

CHOOSE A SHOE THAT SUPPORTS YOUR FEET

When choosing an everyday shoe, check that the fabric or structure around your heel and lower ankle is rigid and provides some support to your foot. This is not only good for comfort, but it also supports your ankle and ensures better posture. If you're looking for an occasion shoe this isn't such a concern, as you won't be wearing it over prolonged periods of time, so lack of support isn't a big problem.

SHOP IN THE AFTERNOON

Your feet swell throughout the day and tend to be their largest in the afternoon. If you shop for shoes in the afternoon, you're more likely to pick a pair that will be comfortable throughout the day.

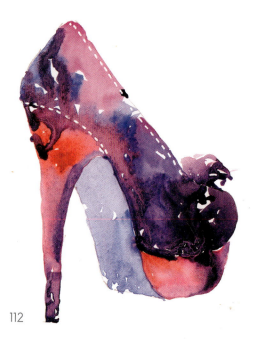

BRING SOCKS

If you're trying on a pair of shoes or boots that you're going to wear with socks or tights but aren't wearing any that day, take some shopping with you. I've bought shoes in the past with tights on and got them home to realise they are just that tiny bit too small when I put my socks on.

TAKE A WALK

It might be a little embarrassing, but there is a reason you were made to walk around the shoe shop as a child before buying new school shoes. If you can't walk in them, or if they are uncomfortable to walk in, they will most likely always be uncomfortable. Yes, natural fabrics do stretch to a certain extent, but they aren't going to transform into a different shoe.

HOW HIGH IS TOO HIGH?

There's an easy way to test if a heel really is too high for you. When you have them on, try to balance on your tiptoes. If your heels lift off the back of the shoe, they are fine. If your heels don't move, they are too high for you and you won't be able to walk properly in them.

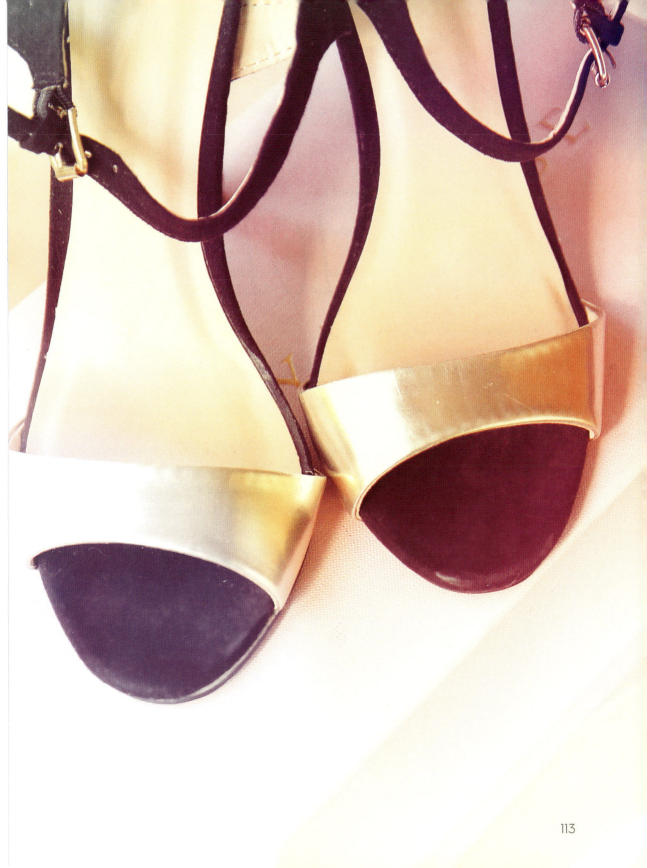

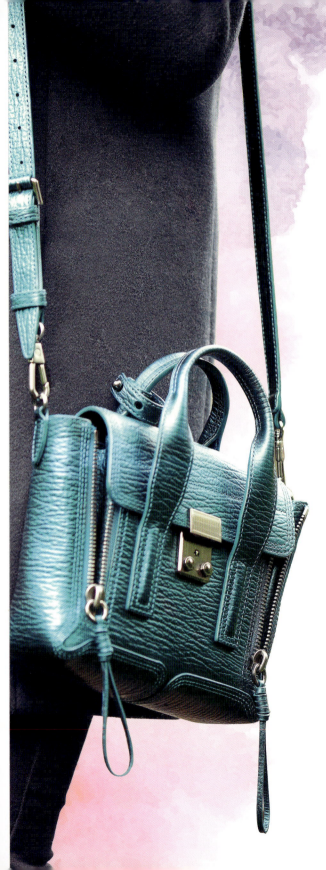

Hazardous Contents

Store makeup, pens and any other potentially staining items in separate pouches in your bag. This will help to prevent the lining from becoming marked (in really bad cases marks may show through to the outside, so this is especially important for larger liquid items like foundation). It'll also make your life easier when it comes to finding things and will make switching handbags quick and stress-free!

Cleaning

To keep your bag in top condition and make it last longer, you should clean it regularly. I switch my handbags over quite frequently, and I always give them a clean before putting them away. I clean the inside by either emptying it upside down in my garden or gently vacuuming it with the brush attachment of my hoover. Depending on the material, you can also wipe the inside and outside of the bag with a slightly damp, clean microfibre cloth. If you have a mark that a damp cloth won't shift, you can try an oil-free baby wipe. Avoid doing this on suede, canvas, untreated or light-coloured bags and always do a small patch test beforehand to make sure it won't mark the material.

Leather Emergencies

I've had my fair share of handbag emergencies over the years. My car keys puncturing a can of Red Bull in my brand-new Mulberry was probably my all-time favourite freak-out moment! But I've always managed to rescue the situation. Whether it's a biro mark, oil spill or general discolouration from wear and tear, there are some incredible restoration services out there. They can be pricey, but if you've invested in a designer bag, they can do an incredible job of bringing even the most tired leather back to life. You can Google a specialist near you by searching for 'handbag leather repair' or 'leather doctor'.

Storage

Storing your handbags carefully when they are not in use will extend their lifetime immensely. It's always best to store them in a dark, dry place. If they come with a dust bag, use it. If they don't, an old pillowcase will do nicely. I also like to stuff mine when not in use, so that they keep their shape. It's best to use bubble wrap if you can, as this will last the longest and won't attract moths. Also try to give them enough space, so they don't get squashed while in storage.

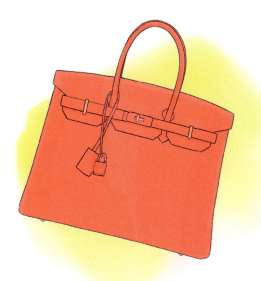

What's In My Handbag?

Night Bag

Lip gloss, concealer and eyeliner: All you need for on-the-go top-ups to keep yourself looking camera–ready.

Breath mints: Chewing gum is not a good look at a classy event.

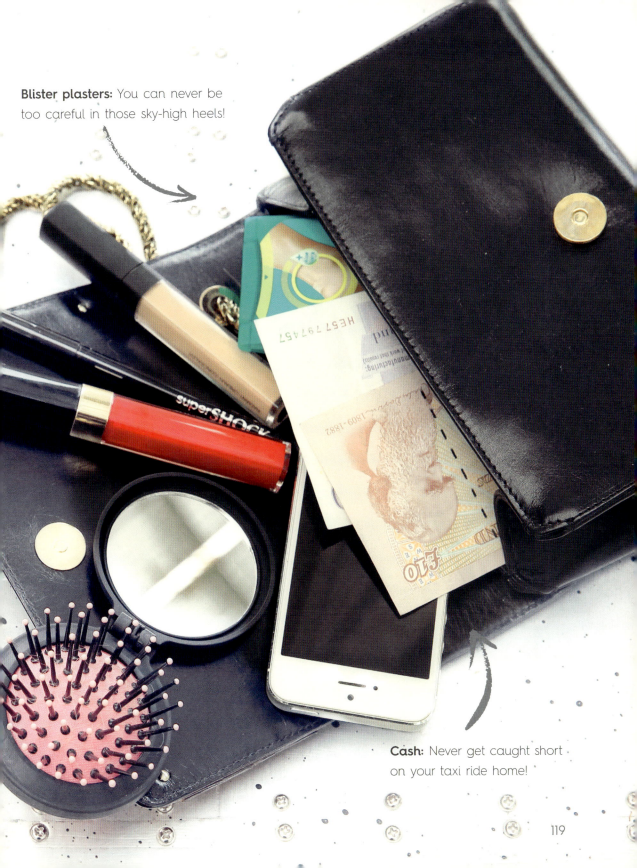

Blister plasters: You can never be too careful in those sky-high heels!

Cash: Never get caught short on your taxi ride home!

119

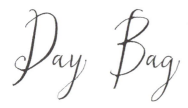

Day Bag

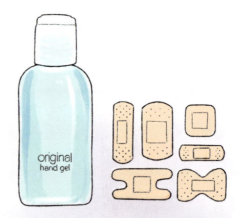

- **Headphones:** Essential for train journeys or working on the go.

- **Kindle**

- **Portable battery pack and phone charger:** My phone battery only lasts half a day at best (too much Twitter?).

- **Blister plasters:** Especially important if you're wearing new shoes!

- **Painkillers**

- **Hand sanitiser:** A public transport must-have!

- **Tampons**

- **Notebook and pen:** For moments of inspiration.

- **Lip gloss, concealer and eyeliner:** My perfect top-up trio! If you get oily, don't forget a compact powder too.

- **Miniature hairbrush and a mirror.**

- **Miniature hairspray**

- **Perfume atomiser:** My favourite is from Travalo. You can fill it with up to 60 sprays of your favourite scent without having to faff around with decanting it from the big bottle.

- **Umbrella:** the smaller the better!

- **Wallet, keys and phone**

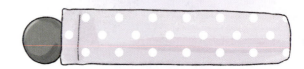

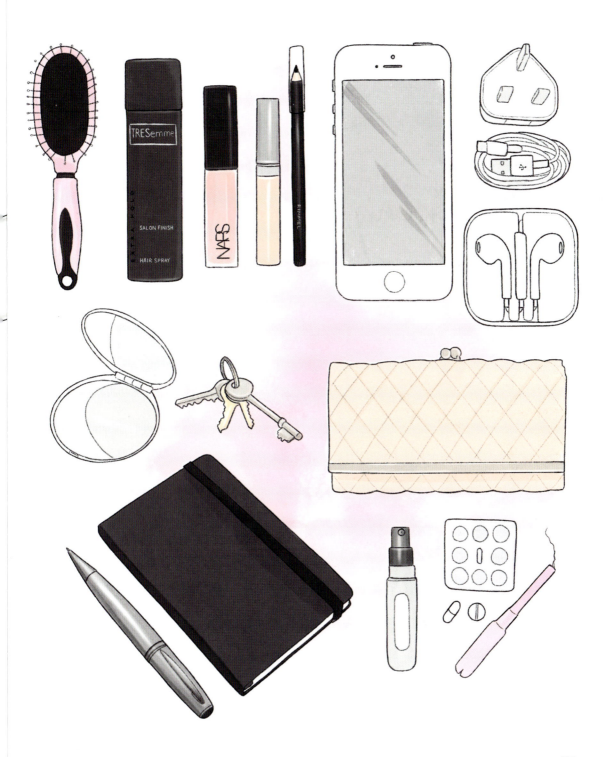

DRESS FOR YOUR SHAPE

Knowing what suits your individual body shape is key when it comes to making the best choices to flatter your figure. Once you've worked out what suits you, you'll also be able to save a lot of time when you're shopping for clothes. The easiest way to work out what you should be wearing and what you should avoid like the fashion plague is to think about which features you consider to be your assets, and which you'd rather not showcase. Accentuate your favourite features by drawing attention to them using colour and cleverly placed accessories. Conceal areas you're less comfortable with in darker shades, loose-fitting fabrics and forgiving textures.

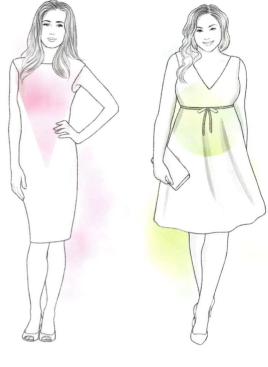

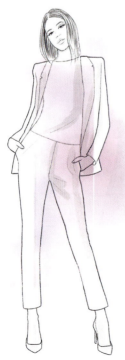

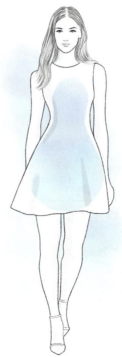

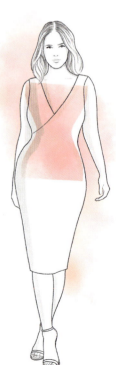

TRY A SIZE UP

If something just doesn't fit right, swallow your pride and try a size up. It may be a bit depressing, but slightly loose clothing is sometimes more flattering than tight, form-fitting items. It depends on the style and cut, but it's always worth trying if you really love an item of clothing but it's not the most flattering to your figure.

USE PRINT AND TEXTURE AS CAMOUFLAGE

Wearing prints and textured fabrics can help to camouflage any areas you don't feel comfortable showing off, but still make a feature of them. Avoid oversized prints however, as these can often have the opposite effect, making you look larger than you actually are.

FLATTERING FABRICS

Fabric is the backbone of any item of clothing. It affects comfort, durability, laundry requirements and, most importantly, the fit. Unforgiving fabrics can turn a perfectly flattering garment into something that accentuates every flaw. Ribbed cotton and lycra are always best avoided if you don't have a washboard stomach. Opt for heavier or knitted fabrics instead, which are more rigid and won't accentuate any lumps and bumps. Silk is also great for concealing any worrisome features and is one of the most comfortable formal fabrics to wear, as it's made of natural fibre.

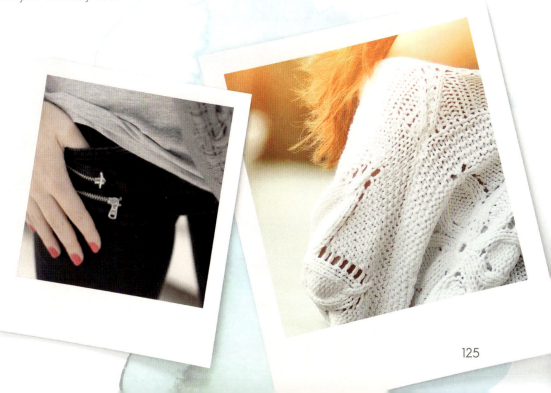

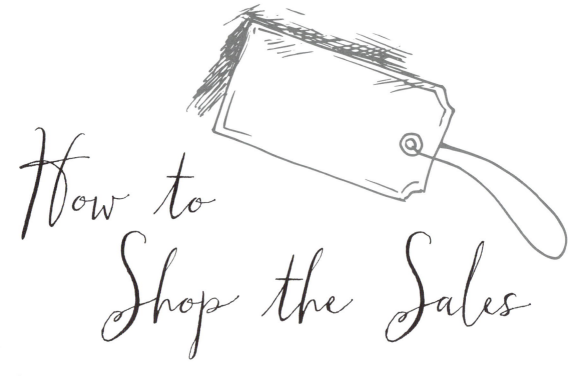

How to Shop the Sales

Sales can be stressful places. You can often come away feeling regretful over not buying something, or wasting money on things you don't really need, but there's nothing more thrilling when it comes to shopping than finding an incredible bargain. Having been a sales addict since my early teens, here's what I've learnt when it comes to bagging the best bargains and enjoying the experience at the same time!

THINK AHEAD

Most shops start their sales online first. As there are no opening hours online, take a quick look on the websites of your favourite shops before you head to the store. This will give you an idea of which items are going to be on sale. You also sometimes see different prices online, so it will help you to truly get the best bargains.

GET THERE EARLY

I'm not one who queues up before the shops open on the first day of the sales, but there is something to be said for getting there early. Not only will you have a better selection to choose from, but everything will be laid out neatly, there won't be as many people struggling to get into the shops and you might actually be able to bag a parking space without queuing for half an hour!

COMFORT IS KEY

Dress for the occasion by wearing your most comfortable shoes and clothing that can easily be removed to make trying on outfits less time-consuming. If it's cold outside, choose a lightweight coat, as chances are it will be sweltering in the shops, and you don't want to be lugging around a bulky coat on top of your finds! No one deals well with pushing, shoving and long queues on an empty stomach either. Make sure you've eaten before you hit the shops. It's also a good idea to take a snack and small bottle of water in your bag, just in case.

HAVE A STRATEGY

Have an idea of where you want to go and what you want to buy. Think about the location of the shops you want to hit, and the potential weight of the bags you might come out with, leaving the heaviest till last if possible.

SET YOURSELF A BUDGET

It's easy to get carried away in the sales and come away with a majorly dented credit card. Avoid shopping guilt by setting a rough budget before you set off, and sticking to it!

TRY THINGS ON

If the queues are ridiculously long you may be tempted to skip this, but if you do, make sure the shop has a good returns policy on their sale items. If you can get to the changing rooms, trying things on can save you from wasting a big chunk of your shopping budget on something that doesn't look absolutely fabulous. You never know, if you have to return something, the second choice item might not be there by the time you go back and you'll have lost your chance.

BE RUTHLESS

Try to avoid buying items simply because they are discounted. Shops love to splash around slogans like 'It's almost free,' but if you don't *love* it, don't buy it. I've spent money on 'ahhh-mazing', hugely discounted sale bargains in the past that I've only worn a couple of times. Even though they are reduced, if you don't wear them as much as the non-sale versions, it's a waste of money.

How to Look Good in a Photo

Everyone wants to look their best in photos. Some people just seem to be naturally more photogenic than others, but there are some tips and tricks you can follow to make sure you look your very best in every picture.

THINK ABOUT YOUR MAKEUP

If you know there are going to be pictures taken with a flash, make sure you choose a foundation with little or no SPF, as makeup with SPF can cause 'flashback' and make your face look ghostly white! It's also really important to choose the perfect shade of foundation (see page 20 to find out how) as tones that are too light or too dark will show up even more on camera. Also, try to avoid glitter or a lot of shimmer in your makeup, as this usually doesn't translate well in photos.

DETERMINE YOUR 'BEST ANGLE'

Take a closer look at the pictures you like most of yourself and look for a recurring pattern in the angles or poses. Once you learn what your best side and most flattering pose is, try to remember it for future picture-taking! To make your face look thinner and your chin more defined, elongate your neck slightly, and angle your chin down a touch – but not back, this will give you a double chin! If you tend to blink in photos, shut your eyes for a couple of seconds before the photo is taken, eliminating the need to blink during the photo. If you're on the end of a group photo, put your hand on your hip and angle your elbow backwards. This will make your arms appear slimmer.

DON'T SLOUCH!

Good posture can make you look both slimmer and more confident. Straighten your spine and pull your shoulders back a little for a more flattering shot. Arranging your body at an angle to the camera lens is also flattering. Try not to align your shoulders straight on with the camera.

BE CONFIDENT!

If you feel awkward posing and having your photo taken, try holding something. A drink, handbag or gift (if it's a party) in hand can help you look and feel a little more relaxed.

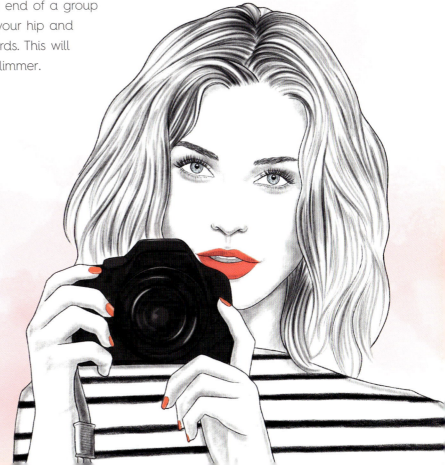

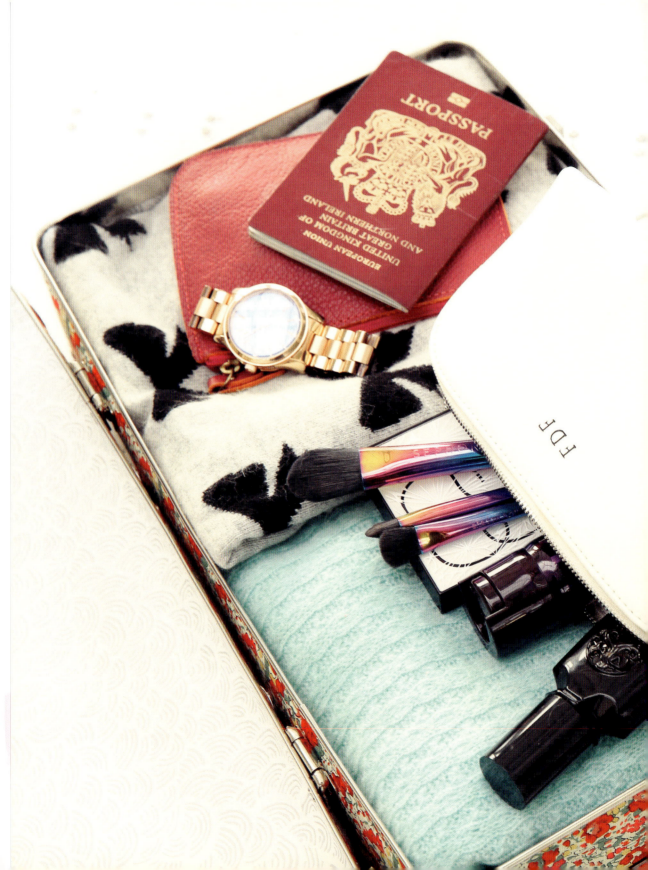

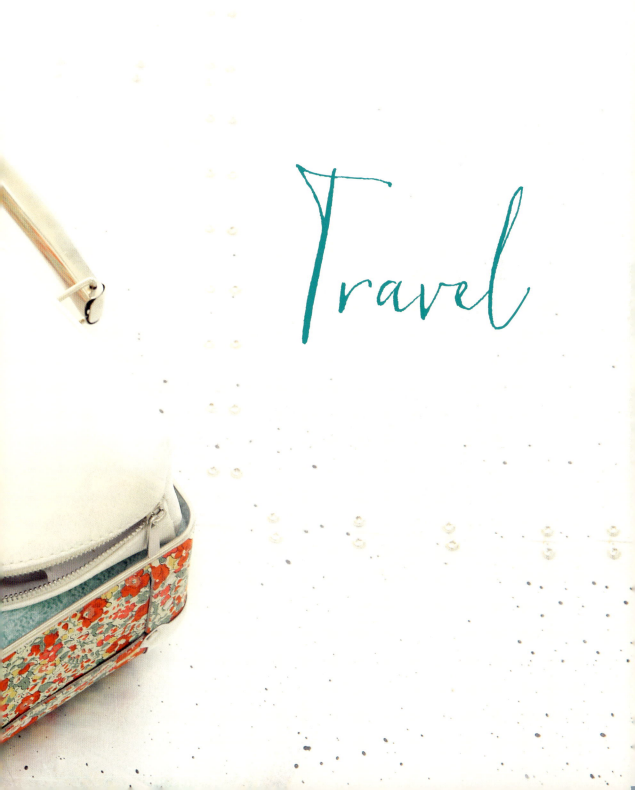

Travel

How to Pack Like a Pro

The process of packing can be a stressful one. After many a long-haul flight, I've pretty much perfected the art of packing just the right amount, while still leaving enough space for potential purchases, and never, ever exceeding the weight limit. Here are my top tips for packing like a pro.

CHECK YOUR WEIGHT ALLOWANCE

Make sure you know what your airline's weight and size restrictions are before you start packing. If you tend to overpack, use the most lightweight suitcase you can find, as this will give you a bit of a head start when it comes to weight limits.

Tip: Invest in a portable luggage scale to make sure you never get charged for excess baggage again. They are cheap to buy and very light and compact. I use mine to weigh my case before leaving for the airport, but also take it with me for the return flight too.

DECIDE WHAT YOU WANT TO PACK IN ADVANCE

Make a list of everything you need to pack and lay it out so you can see it all together. I like to lay out entire outfits I think I might want to wear and try to put together a 'capsule' wardrobe that works for the amount of time I'm away for. If all of the items can be worn together in various different combinations, you'll be able to create a lot of different looks with fewer items of clothing. Don't forget to make a separate list while you're packing of things you need to remember to throw in at the last minute (your phone charger, hair dryer, toothbrush etc.). Go through your checklist before you leave for the airport, to double check you haven't forgotten any essentials!

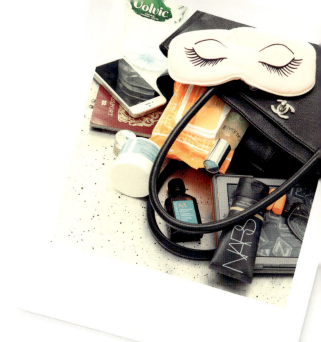

Tip: Never put essential or valuable items in your check-in baggage. Keep them on you at all times. You never know when your bag might go missing, or be left unattended and vulnerable to thieves taking a peek inside!

MAKE THE MOST OF YOUR SPACE

Rolling your clothes instead of folding them is a great way to minimise the space they take up in your suitcase and to reduce creasing too. It's good to do this if you have an unstructured suitcase or duffel bag, but may not be suitable for certain items of clothing. If a garment is made of soft, thick fabric that doesn't crease easily, like jeans and T-shirts, rolling is great. Avoid rolling thinner, more delicate fabrics that crease easily, like silk. If you have a structured suitcase and more delicate clothing, fold your items neatly, along seams if you can, to minimise creasing. Another great tip to avoid creases when folding your clothes is to fold numerous items together. This makes each fold thicker, so the fabric is 'bending' instead of creasing.

Fill shoes with jewellery or belts. This will not only save space, but will offer some protection for your jewellery too. You'll probably want to put jewellery in a travel pouch beforehand; the little pouches you sometimes get with high-end makeup are great for this. Fill any leftover shoe space with socks. Pack heavy items along the wheelbase, or at the bottom of your suitcase. This will make sure they don't squash, compress or crease the other items in your case.

Don't forget to pack your underwear in a separate zipped section of your bag, to ensure you don't have any embarrassing experiences if your luggage splits open or gets searched!

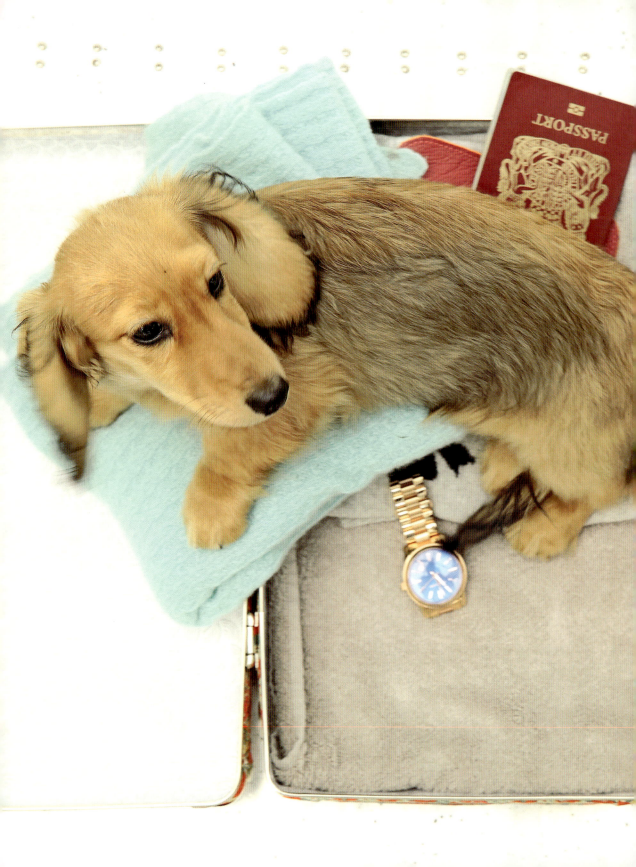

TRAVEL-SIZED TOILETRIES AREN'T JUST FOR YOUR CARRY-ON

I try to miniaturise as much of my wash bag as I can. This means you can take more items with you, to cover any beauty or hair eventuality, but it also saves space on the way home, as you are likely to have finished the small bottles and can dispose of them (and make more space for souvenirs!). Also make sure you pack your toiletries in a plastic bag to protect the rest of your luggage in case something leaks. I put my entire wash bag in a plastic bag, so it's quick and easy to unpack upon arrival.

CONSIDER WHAT YOU MIGHT BUY ON YOUR TRIP

If you're going somewhere where you are likely to buy a few items of clothing, you may have to pack less. If you want to do a lot of shopping, pack a collapsible case or duffel bag, as checking in another bag is often cheaper than paying hefty excess baggage charges when you get to the airport!

Tip: If you want to use a lock on your luggage, make sure it's government-approved. Otherwise the authorities will use force to open it if they need to, and could end up damaging your luggage.

Travelling in Style

Choosing the right outfit to travel in can change your in-flight experience more than you'd expect. I have something of an onboard uniform. Here are my tips for travelling in style without compromising on comfort.

AVOID TRACKSUITS IN THE AIRPORT

While you want to be comfortable, dressing too casually will dash any chance of getting upgraded and will leave you looking scruffy upon arrival. If you do want to wear a tracksuit or onesie onboard, pack it in your carry-on bag and get changed just before you get on the plane, and again just before you get off. I usually go for some stretchy jeans or leggings, a big hoody and some fluffy socks for keeping warm and cosy on the plane.

PACK A CHANGE OF CLOTHES

Whether or not I'm changing into something more comfortable for the plane journey itself, I always pack a fresh set of clothes to put on when I disembark a long-haul flight. This is especially important if I'm meeting people at the airport, or going straight to an engagement, as it's the best way to ensure you leave the plane looking fresh, clean and crease-free. Layering is also a great way to ensure you have the appropriate clothing for both your origin and destination without having to haul too many clothes in your carry-on. It's usually cold on the plane so layering makes sure you are prepared for all temperatures.

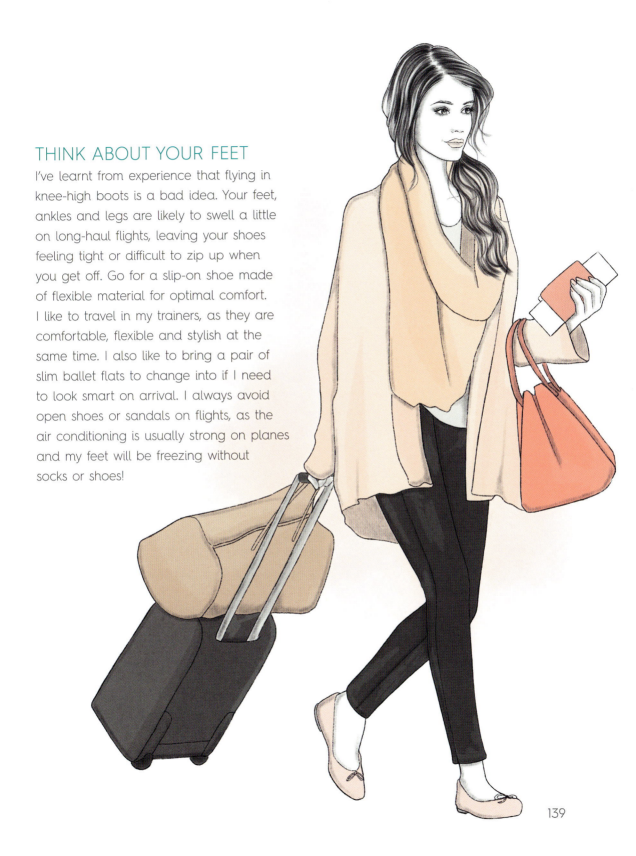

THINK ABOUT YOUR FEET

I've learnt from experience that flying in knee-high boots is a bad idea. Your feet, ankles and legs are likely to swell a little on long-haul flights, leaving your shoes feeling tight or difficult to zip up when you get off. Go for a slip-on shoe made of flexible material for optimal comfort. I like to travel in my trainers, as they are comfortable, flexible and stylish at the same time. I also like to bring a pair of slim ballet flats to change into if I need to look smart on arrival. I always avoid open shoes or sandals on flights, as the air conditioning is usually strong on planes and my feet will be freezing without socks or shoes!

139

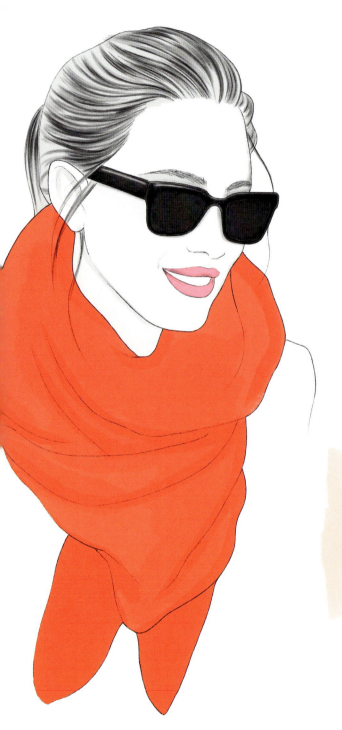

BRING YOUR BIGGEST, WARMEST SCARF

Even if it's mid-summer, I always take a big, soft scarf on long-haul flights, as it comes in handy for so many things. Whether it's for a makeshift neck pillow, regular pillow, blanket or shawl for covering your face while you sleep, you won't regret bringing it along!

DARK SUNGLASSES ARE ESSENTIAL

They can hide even the most tired eyes, and look stylish at the same time! Wearing them on the plane is totally OTT, but they are a must-have for early-morning departures or long-haul arrivals.

Tip: Invest in good-quality luggage. Not only will it last longer than a cheap suitcase, you'll also look more stylish when using it. I've collected my set of leather luggage over a seven-year period, and even after many long-haul flights and a lot of mishandling by airlines, it only gets better with age.

In-Flight Beauty

When I first started taking long-haul flights, I did nothing with my skin, then started to wonder why it always looked dry and uneven for a few days after I landed. Time and experience has taught me the hard way how important a long-haul skincare routine is, especially if you want to look fabulous for the duration of your trip. Follow my in-flight beauty tips for beautiful skin on arrival and return!

WASH YOUR HANDS

Either in the bathroom before boarding or using hand-sanitiser, you'll want to make sure your hands are clean before touching your face. It's also advisable to use hand-sanitiser every few hours onboard, to keep germs at bay.

REMOVE YOUR MAKEUP

Face wipes are the best option for this (Ole Henriksen make the best ones, but Simple are also good if you're on a budget). Even if you're not wearing makeup, you should still make sure your skin is clean before applying anything else.

APPLY AN INTENSIVE MOISTURISER

You want to choose a product that will not only nourish your skin, but also work as a barrier against the drying effects of the onboard air conditioning. Apply a thick layer of your favourite night cream, or use a thicker cream like Elizabeth Arden's Eight Hour Cream or Weleda's Skin Food. I top mine up two or three times throughout longer flights. You can also apply an overnight mask. These are basically intensive treatments that sink into your skin, so you can leave them on for an extended period of time without scaring the cabin crew! My favourite one for flying is the First Aid Beauty Facial Radiance overnight mask, but Clinique also make a good one. Sheet masks are also great for flights, but a bit more high maintenance, as you have to dispose of them after use, and they also look a bit ridiculous!

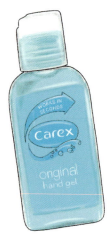

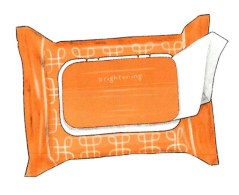

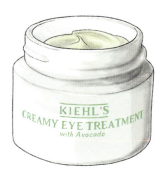

DON'T FORGET YOUR EYES

The combination of lack of sleep, air conditioning and jet lag is not good for the under-eye situation! Don't forget to treat your eyes to a rich eye cream at least once during your flight (Kiehl's Creamy Avocado eye cream is perfect for this). Also have a de-puffing, cooling eye-gel rollerball on hand for when you land (I love the Drops of Youth one from The Body Shop).

LIPS AND HANDS

Two more essential products I never board without are lip balm and hand cream. My lips always dry out on flights, so I often use my Eight Hour Cream on my lips as well as my face. Pack a miniature version of your favourite hand cream to keep your mitts nicely hydrated.

HAIR MAINTENANCE

Your hair is an asset that often gets forgotten in the sky. Some people recommend putting a leave-in conditioner onto dry hair in-flight, but this will leave you looking greasy on arrival. Go for a little hair oil (Moroccan Oil is my favourite) and massage a drop into the lengths and ends of your hair every three or four hours to stop it looking frazzled. A portable hairbrush also makes a useful addition if you want to look polished when you land.

H_2O

One of the most important aspects of in-flight skincare is to keep hydrated. Combat the effects of the moisture-sucking air conditioning by drinking a litre of water for every five hours you spend in the air.

Tip: Don't forget you can only carry on liquid, cream and gel products up to 100ml (or 3.4oz) in your hand luggage. Check all of your beauty products beforehand, so they don't have to be thrown away at security.

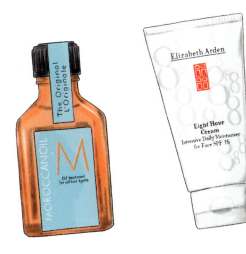

How to Beat Jet Lag

Jet lag is one of the most frustrating things about travelling. When you're really excited to be away on holiday and have a jam-packed schedule of things to do, the last thing you need is to be awake all night and feeling like a zombie all day long. I used to suffer really badly with jet lag when travelling long haul, but now I have a strict routine to help me minimise its effects and to get over the time difference. Fast. Here are my secrets.

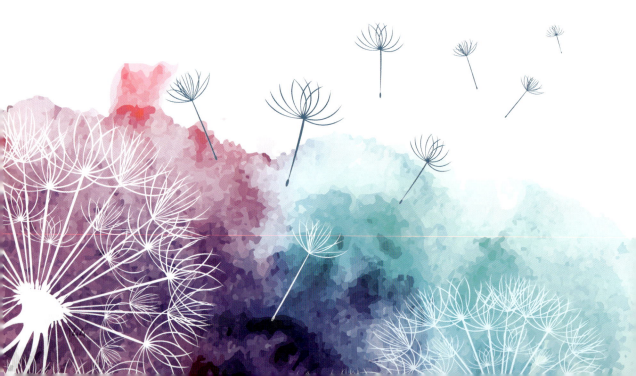

BEFORE YOU LEAVE

Adjust your sleeping patterns if you can. If you're travelling east, try to go to bed an hour *earlier* than normal for three consecutive nights before you fly. If heading west, an hour *later*.

Take care of yourself. You'll bounce back from jet lag more quickly if you are in good health, stress-free and generally well-rested before you travel. Try to eat well and hit the gym a few times the week before you leave.

Download an app. There are loads of jet lag management apps available now, and a lot of them are free. Download one onto your phone to help you work out when you're meant to be sleeping and eating, both before, during and after your trip.

Pack a travel pillow, earplugs and an eye mask. These are three essentials I never, ever travel without. If you want to get some sleep on the plane, these will double your chances!

IN-FLIGHT

Change your watch to the time at your destination as soon as you board the plane. This will leave you less confused and help you get your head around the time difference from the get-go. It will also help you know when you should and shouldn't be sleeping. If it's daytime at your destination, try to stay awake during the flight. If it's nighttime, try your best to get some sleep.

Food also plays a big part in your sleep cycle, so try to eat at the 'right' times for your destination, adjusting your meal times as soon as you get on the plane.

Drink lots of water. Dehydration can mess with your system and make jet lag even worse. Sip on water throughout your flight to keep hydrated. This is also great for your skin.

Avoid alcohol, caffeine and junk food on the plane, as all of these will affect your body's natural sleep cycle. Taking your own meal and healthy snacks onto the plane is a good idea if you want to steer clear of junk food. A lot of plane food is high in fat and salt, so planning ahead and buying some healthier options in the airport before you fly is a smart idea.

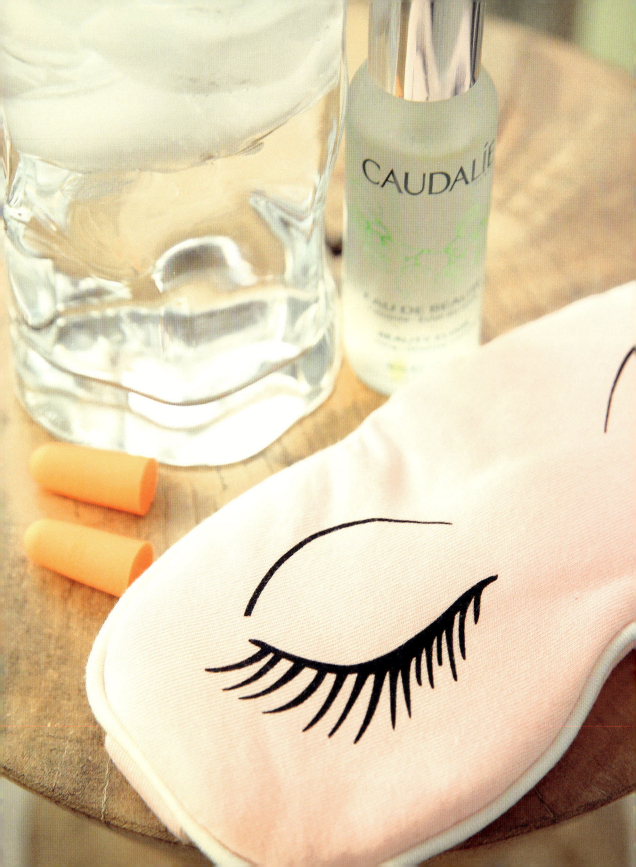

WHEN YOU ARRIVE

Stick to a schedule. If you arrive in the morning, don't go to sleep! No matter how tempting it is to take a 'quick' afternoon nap to satiate your senses, try to stay awake until at least 10 p.m. local time, to start kicking the jet lag from the get-go.

If you suffer really badly with jet lag, you can get sleeping pills over the counter at your local pharmacist before you leave, or you can opt for a natural melatonin pill to help you get to sleep and stay asleep all night. Avoid strong prescription sleeping pills, as you won't be gradually adjusting your natural sleep cycle as much as knocking yourself out. I take melatonin for the first three nights of my trip if I'm going somewhere with more than five hours' time difference.

Expose yourself to natural light at the right times. Sunlight is a strong stimulant for our body clocks. Getting outside into the sunshine will help your body adjust to the time difference more quickly. Exercise also helps your body to regulate itself more quickly, so try going for a brisk walk, hike or getting into the gym in the morning to wake yourself up.

Continue to avoid alcohol, caffeine and junk food. This might be tricky if you're on holiday, but it's best to avoid these if you can, as they affect your body's natural sleep cycle and can cause dehydration.

It's likely that people at home who don't know you're away will try to call you when you're asleep. Put your phone on silent to avoid being woken up. Once you're awake, it's hard to doze off again if your body thinks it's daytime at home.

Set an alarm. This is especially important when travelling east, as your body will want to stay asleep in the morning. When the alarm goes off force yourself to get up and outside. A protein-rich breakfast (eggs and avocado is my personal favourite) will help to wake you up. Avoid eating a sugary breakfast, as that will only give you a temporary spike in energy.

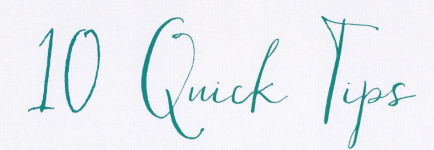

10 Quick Tips

Block the Noise

Never (ever!) forget earplugs on long-haul flights, or when staying in a hotel. You never know how noisy it will be, or if you'll be seated next to a crying baby.

Get Comfortable

Invest in an expensive neck pillow if you travel a lot. The cheaper ones don't give you as much support and wear out more quickly. The best ones are made of memory foam.

Keep Feet Toasty

Pack some fuzzy socks in your carry-on when flying long haul. Most airlines have stopped providing free socks in economy class now. These will keep your feet warm and ensure you can leave your shoes off for the entire flight.

Do Your Research

Read online reviews before you book! This one might be obvious, but no matter how amazing a hotel looks on its own website, I always exhaust the TripAdvisor website before I choose somewhere to stay. This way, you can ensure you are getting the best possible location, quality and service within your budget.

Get Covered

Don't forget to buy travel insurance. It's not very expensive and is a total travel essential. Hopefully you won't need it, but if you do and have taken the risk of not getting it, you will live to regret it!

Passport Protection

Keep a copy of your passport either on your phone or in your luggage. It's a traveller's worst nightmare to lose their passport, but if you do lose it, having a copy will speed up the process of getting a replacement.

Keep Info to Hand

Take the address of your hotel and any booking confirmations in your carry-on luggage. This sounds obvious, but a lot of people keep this information in their emails or checked-in luggage. You usually need to include this information on your landing card and won't normally have access to wifi upon arrival.

Switch off Your Roaming

Switch off your data roaming as soon as you get on the plane, before you turn your phone off. This will stop any extra data charges that you may inadvertently get if you only switch it off after you've landed.

Book the Best Seat

Reserve your seat before you fly! If your airline offers this free of charge, make sure you choose a seat before you fly, as this can affect your in-flight experience hugely. If you're on a long-haul flight, think about where you would be happiest. If it's an overnight flight, I always prefer to be in an aisle seat, so that I can get to the toilet without waking people up. I also try to get a seat as close to the front of the plane as possible, as it usually means you'll be able to get off first. If you're bothered by bad smells (who isn't?) try to get a seat a good distance away from the toilets! Websites like SeatGuru and SeatExpert will help you choose the best seats available.

Nervous Flyer?

Check the aeroplane model and layout before booking. I always keep an eye on which model of aircraft I'm booking onto. If you're a nervous flyer, avoid smaller planes for long-haul flights, as they are more prone to turbulence. I also Google pictures of the airline's interior of each specific model and try to work out how old the plane is to ensure the cleanest, most comfortable and high-tech in-flight experience possible!

Health

and Fitness

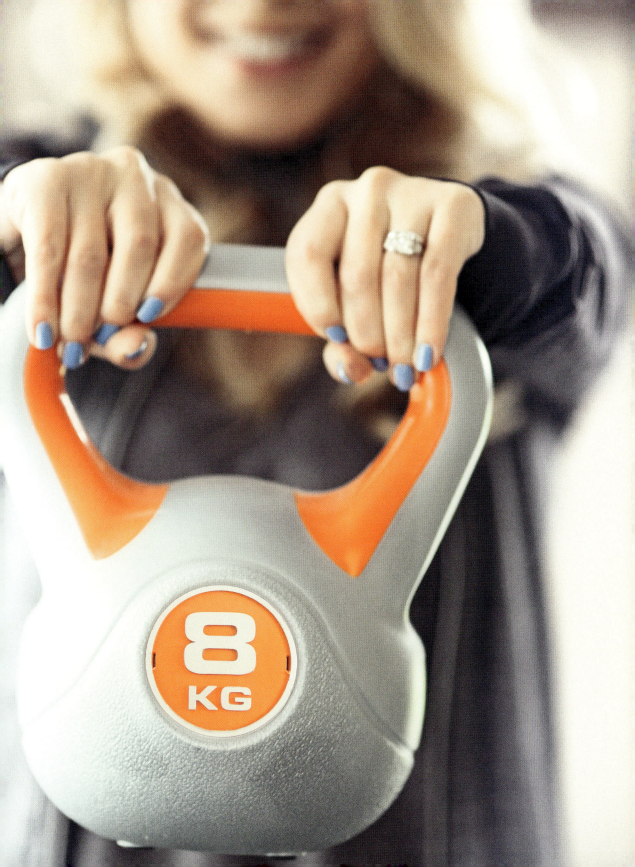

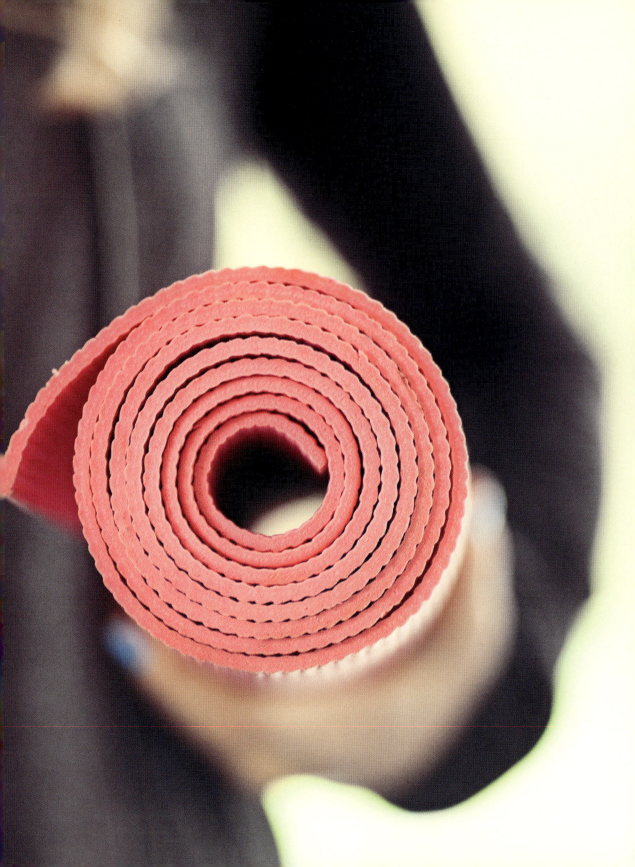

Introduction

While it's easy to concern yourself with the superficial side of looking good, it's important to remember that looking after yourself is essential not only for looking your best but also feeling your best. Eating well and looking after your body has obvious health benefits, but most of the time you'll notice a difference in the way you *feel* about yourself too. It's important to highlight that when I talk about being fit and healthy, I'm *not* talking about losing weight or eating less. Weight loss can be a side effect of making changes to your current lifestyle, but essentially it's all about being aware of what you put into your body, how you look after it and also the positive implications a healthier lifestyle can have on your energy levels and overall health and happiness.

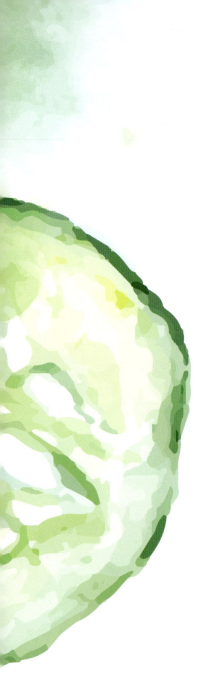

Skin Food

'You are what you eat', as they say, and food really can have an impact on your skin, both good and bad. Your choice of food can make a big difference to breakouts, inflammation, sun damage and even wrinkle formation. I've put together a list of the goodies and baddies when it comes to your skin.

THE GOODIES

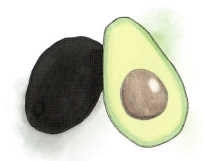

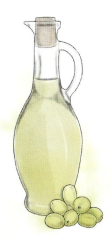

Avocado

Rich in fatty acids, vitamins and antioxidants, avocados can help to minimise environmental damage that causes fine lines and wrinkles, including sun damage. They also contain vitamin C, which is good for encouraging the production of elastin and collagen in the skin and can also help to boost skin hydration.

Olive Oil

Great for skin hydration. Contrary to popular belief, olive oil is not brilliant for cooking with, as it degrades very easily when exposed to heat and light. Save your best extra virgin olive oil for drizzling over salads and vegetables or adding to dips and dressings.

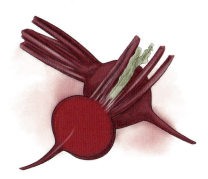

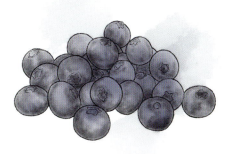

Beetroot

A natural anti-ageing treatment, beetroot is high in folate, which naturally helps to stimulate the production and repair of cells. It can also help to reduce skin inflammation.

Blueberries

Packed with antioxidants and vitamins that fight the free radicals that accelerate ageing, they can also help boost the elasticity of the skin and help to strengthen blood vessels to avoid broken capillaries.

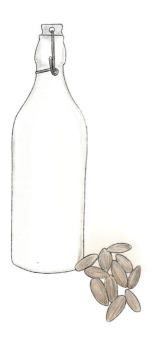

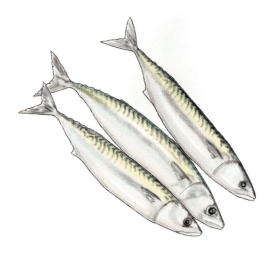

Almond Milk

Not only a great alternative to dairy, almond milk is also packed with vitamin E, which can help boost skin hydration.

Oily Fish

Eating oily fish like salmon, sardines and mackerel, which contain omega-3 fatty acids, can help delay the ageing process. Not only do they strengthen your cell membranes, protecting your skin against damaging free radicals and breakouts, but they also reduce inflammation and help with skin conditions like eczema and psoriasis.

THE BADDIES

Caffeine

Causes an increase in the body's stress hormone cortisol, which can lead to increased wrinkle formation (and belly fat!).

Alcohol

Can disrupt your hormones and liver, causing breakouts, and reduce blood flow to the skin, leaving it looking dull, especially if you binge drink.

Refined Sugar

Steals hydration from your skin and can help accelerate the ageing process. It's very hard to cut it out entirely, but if you want to see a significant improvement in your skin you should definitely eat it in moderation.

Dairy

Dairy has long been linked to acne, but rather than cutting it out entirely, it's more important to think about the *type* of dairy you are eating. Non-organic dairy produce can disrupt your hormones (due to the hormones that are given to the animals) and result in breakouts, so it's best to stick to good quality, organic dairy produce.

Fried Food

Bad for your body and skin. A great alternative is to 'healthy fry' your food using an air fryer. This uses a tiny amount of oil, but still produces tasty fried food – even chips!

Fizzy Drinks

Have been linked to premature ageing. If you're tempted to reach for the diet version, artificial sweeteners can slow down your metabolism, so you're not always making a healthier choice. Choose naturally sweetened soft drinks like Zevia if you still want a fizzy fix.

Gluten

Not everyone is intolerant to gluten, but if you do have problems with your skin, it's worth cutting it out for a few weeks to see if you notice an improvement. A lot of people are only very mildly intolerant, which might not show up in a test, but may well cause issues for your skin.

Overcooked Food

Overcooked or burnt food can accelerate the ageing process and also minimises the nutrients you get from it. Steam, poach or sauté your food instead.

Non-Organic Veg

Toxins from pesticides and chemicals used on non-organic veg are often retained in the flesh. This is transferred to the body when you eat them, and can be detrimental to your skin. They increase the level of free radicals in your system and can limit your skin's natural repair process.

Juices Vs. Smoothies

Making a glass of my own fresh juice in the morning is one of my favourite ways to start the day. As the juicing craze has exploded over the past couple of years, it's easy to get confused about what it is, why it's so good for you, when you should be juicing and how to make the best juices. Here's what I've found works for me.

WHAT'S THE DIFFERENCE?

Juices often get confused with smoothies. The key difference is that a juicer completely separates the juice from the pulp, while smoothies simply blend everything together, leaving in the pulp and therefore all of the insoluble fibre. But which is better? The short answer is: neither. Both are good, but for different reasons.

Juices are made in a juicer, which extracts only the water and 70 per cent of the nutrients from the fruit and vegetables you put in. Although juicing doesn't extract all of the nutrients, the lack of insoluble fibre in the end product means that 100 per cent of these remaining nutrients are absorbed very quickly, without your body having to work hard to digest them. Therefore juices are a great way to pack extra nutrients into your diet and are also a good way to cleanse and detox, as they give your digestive system a break. Juicing high-sugar fruits, however, can give you a spike in blood sugar levels. This is why it's recommended to add lots of vegetables to your juices, and why green juice has become popular over the past few years.

On the other hand, blending leaves in 100 per cent of the insoluble fibre and therefore the nutrients. Fibre is indigestible and essentially just aids the body's natural bowel movements. It makes your smoothie heavy and thick, but also fills you up and your body absorbs the nutrients over a longer period of time. The fibre also inhibits some of the nutrients from being absorbed into the body, so you're not actually able to absorb that missing 30 per cent of the nutrients you lose when juicing.

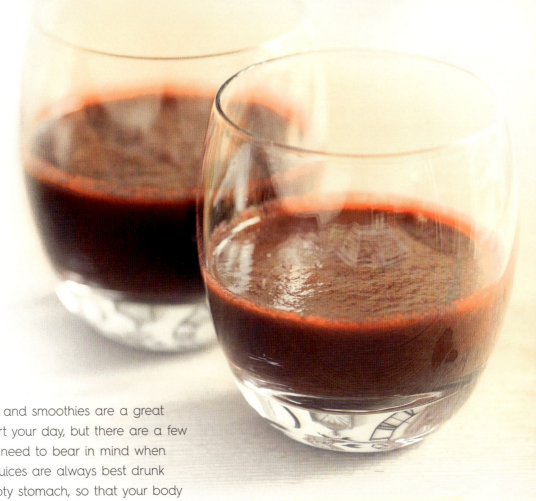

WHEN?

Both juices and smoothies are a great way to start your day, but there are a few things you need to bear in mind when doing so. Juices are always best drunk on an empty stomach, so that your body can get the full benefit. They often aren't filling, though, so I like to make a juice first thing in the morning, then follow it with a small breakfast of eggs or yoghurt 20 minutes later. It's also really important to drink juices and smoothies within 15 minutes of making them. The nutrients will start to degrade as soon as they meet the air, so the longer you leave it before drinking your concoction, the less benefit you'll be getting.

Tip: Clean your juicer or blender straight away after use. If you leave it to dry, the residue is ten times harder to wash off!

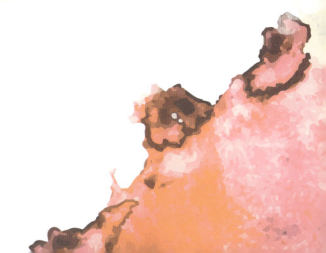

Juice: My Top 3 Recipes

BEETROOT BOOSTER

1 apple
5 kale leaves
½ a beetroot
½ a carrot
½-inch chunk of ginger

Benefits: Beetroot is high in dietary nitrate, which can help to naturally lower blood pressure, while ginger is packed with antioxidants.

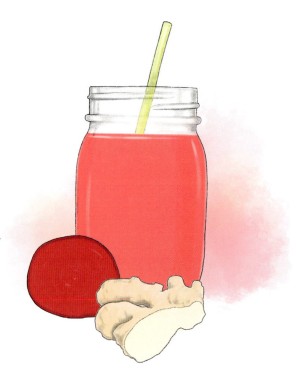

MORE THAN A MOJITO

1 apple
½ a cucumber
1 lime
1 handful of mint leaves

Benefits: Cucumber contains
alkaline-forming minerals that can help to
balance the pH level of your blood. The
skin is also packed with vitamins A and C,
so be sure to juice it whole!

POPEYE

5 handfuls of spinach
1 handful of kale
2 sticks of celery
⅓ of a cucumber
1 apple
½ a lemon
Optional: ½ a jalapeño (for a bit of a kick!)

Benefits: Spinach contains high levels of
vitamin K, along with a long list of other
vitamins, which plays an important role
in your blood's ability to clot and also
encourages the absorption of calcium, so
it's good for keeping your bones and teeth
strong and healthy. The health benefits of
kale are also seemingly endless. It's great
for your blood, skin and muscles, and can
help to lower cholesterol levels.

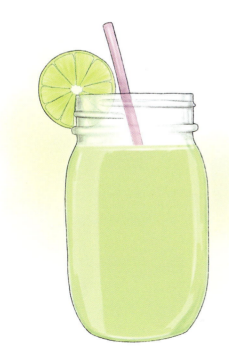

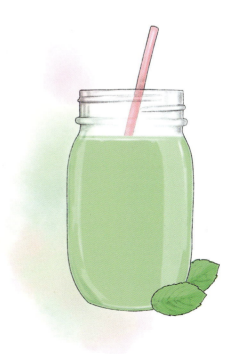

Smoothies: My Top 3 Recipes

THE HULK

¼ of an avocado
1 pear
1 kiwi
2 handfuls of spinach
1 handful of kale

Benefits: The 'good' fat in avocados can help keep your heart healthy. They are also full of anti-inflammatory nutrients and antioxidants, so they're great for your skin and eyes, as well as helping to regulate your blood sugar level.

Tip: Avocado gives a creaminess to your smoothie without having to add dairy.

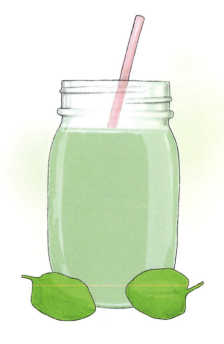

PEANUT POWER

½ a banana

1 cup of milk (skimmed cow's milk, almond milk or coconut milk)

1 tablespoon of peanut butter

1 tablespoon of flaxseed

1 handful of ice

Benefits: Bananas contain high levels of potassium and healthy carbohydrates, so they give you an energy boost that lasts much longer than simple sugars. They are also great for your heart, stomach and digestive system.

SWEET TREAT

1 kiwi

1 handful of frozen strawberries

1 banana

75ml apple juice

Benefits: Kiwis are full of vitamin C, so they're great for your immune system. They are also high in potassium and fibre and can help maintain a healthy heart.

Tip: If you're short of time, try using frozen fruit in your smoothies. It'll save preparation time and mean your smoothies are wonderfully cold without the need for ice.

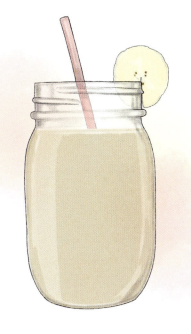

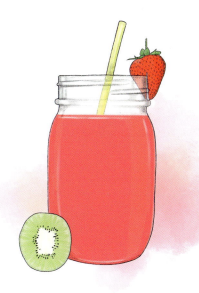

5 Healthy Breakfast Ideas

STRAWBERRY PARFAIT

This sweet treat tastes like a dessert, but is low in calories and fat. It's a good choice for those of you with a sweet tooth who want to find a healthier alternative to sugary breakfasts.

Ingredients

1 pot of fat-free Greek yoghurt
1 teaspoon of Stevia
2 handfuls of strawberries
1 handful of blueberries
2 tablespoons of granola

Add the Stevia (natural sweetener) to your yoghurt and mix it in thoroughly. Cut the strawberries into quarters and mix them with your blueberries. Take a tall glass and add a layer of yoghurt, then a layer of fruit, another of yoghurt, then a tablespoon of granola. Repeat this process and you'll have a perfect, guilt-free strawberry parfait!

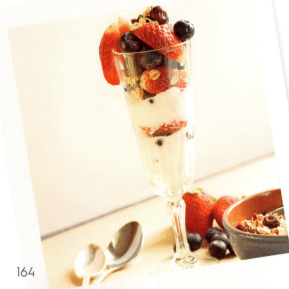

BAKED AVOCADO EGG

There is no better combination than avocado and eggs when it comes to breakfast food! This baked option is filling yet healthy, and makes for a perfect post-workout breakfast choice.

Ingredients

1 large avocado
2 small to medium eggs
chives
chilli flakes, to taste
salt and pepper, to taste

Halve your avocado and remove the stone. Crack an egg into each half and sprinkle over a pinch of chilli flakes and chives (you may have to scoop out a little avocado to make space for the eggs, depending on the size of your avocado and its stone). Put the avocado halves into the oven on a medium heat for 10–15 minutes. The cooking time will depend on the size of your eggs and the avocado, so keep an eye on it until the egg is cooked. Remove from the oven and add salt and pepper to taste.

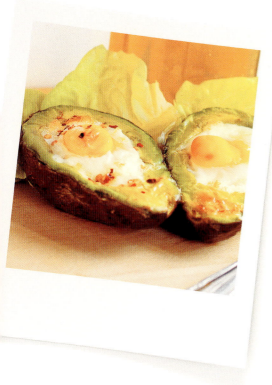

GUILT-FREE CHOCOLATE BANANA BREAD

Banana bread is one of my favourite sweet treats, but it's also perfect for breakfast on the go. Here is my recipe for a wholemeal, guilt-free version made with agave nectar, fat-free yoghurt and cacao nibs for an extra crunch!

Ingredients

140g wholemeal flour
100g self-raising flour
1 teaspoon of bicarbonate of soda
1 teaspoon of baking powder
3 tablespoons of cacao nibs
pinch of salt
3 eggs
300g mashed bananas (preferably over-ripe and blackened)
4 tablespoons of agave nectar
150ml fat-free natural yoghurt

Mix together all of the dry ingredients. In a separate bowl, beat the eggs and combine with all of the wet ingredients. Mix the wet mixture into the dry and pour into a lined and greased bread tin. Bake the mixture for 1 hour and 10 minutes at 160°C or until a knife comes out clean.

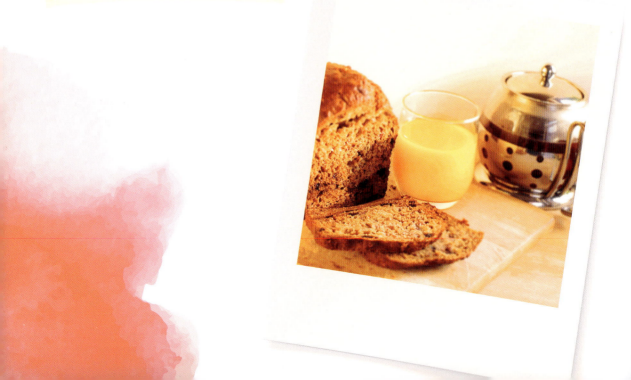

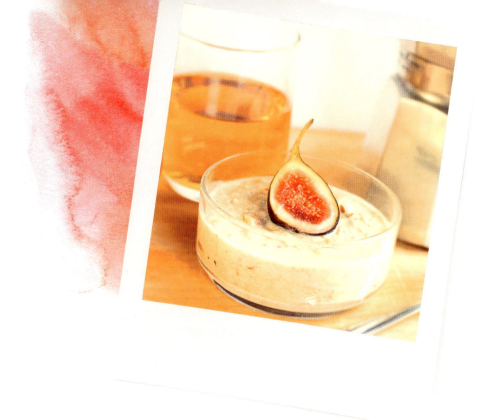

HOMEMADE BIRCHER MUESLI

A fruity spin on normal muesli, Bircher muesli has been around since the early 1900s. There are hundreds of different takes on this Swiss breakfast. This homemade fig and almond version is my favourite.

Ingredients

25g oats
6 tablespoons of apple juice
1 apple
1 handful of almonds
2 tablespoons of fat-free Greek yoghurt
1 fresh fig

Soak the oats in the apple juice overnight. In the morning, grate your apple into the mixture and add your almonds and Greek yoghurt. Mix it all together and top with a chopped fresh fig.

SPINACH AND HAM EGG WRAP

This fun spin on a traditional omelette is quick to make, easy to eat on the go, low in fat and packed with protein.

Ingredients

2 eggs
2 handfuls of spinach
2 slices of ham

Whisk up the eggs and pour them into a non-stick pan. Cook them for about a minute before evenly scattering your spinach over the top. Cover the pan and wait for three to four minutes until the egg is almost cooked. Add your slices of ham and carefully roll the omelette up like a wrap. Cut it in half and eat!

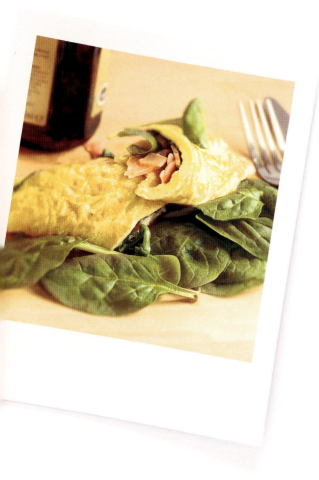

3 Packed Lunch Ideas

RAW KALE SALAD JAR

This is one of my favourite salads to make at home, and it's also a great choice for a packed lunch. Making salads in jars is a great way of keeping them fresh till lunchtime. They key is to layer them up, starting with the dressing at the bottom, then the salad itself, then the toppings. When you're ready to eat it, all you need to do is give it a good shake to combine all of the ingredients and eat it right out of the jar!

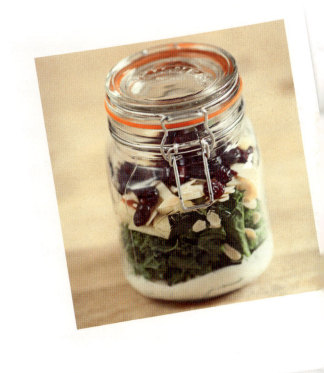

Ingredients

3 tablespoons of ranch dressing (if you want a healthier version, try a balsamic or vinaigrette dressing)
3 large handfuls of raw kale
½ an apple, chopped
1 handful of dried cranberries
1 handful of sliced, toasted almonds

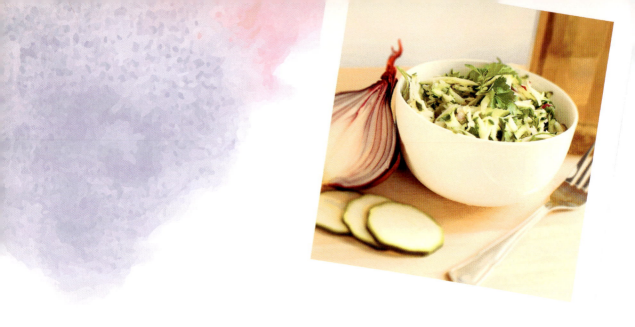

GRATED COURGETTE SALAD

This courgette salad is quick and easy to make but packs a serious punch in the taste department. It makes a nice change from conventional salads, and you can make it more filling by adding a grilled chicken breast or salmon fillet.

Ingredients

1 courgette
1 lemon
1 lime
1 small red onion
1 large handful of coriander
a drizzle of extra virgin olive oil
salt and pepper, to taste

Grate the courgette into a bowl and squeeze the juice of one lemon and one lime over it. Finely chop your red onion, tear up a handful of coriander and combine it all for a fresh and tasty variation on your average salad. Finish it off with a drizzle of olive oil and salt and pepper to taste.

QUINOA STUFFED PEPPERS

These stuffed peppers are delicious hot or cold, and make a great packed lunch if you have a little time to prepare them the night before. Quinoa is packed with protein, so it's a great choice for vegetarians and meat-eaters alike if you want a healthy, low-fat, protein-rich packed lunch.

Ingredients

½ cup of quinoa
1 clove of garlic
1 small onion
1 teaspoon of olive oil
1 medium tomato
1 small handful of basil
1 red pepper
1 handful of grated cheddar cheese
optional: a sprinkle of chilli flakes

Boil your quinoa with a cup of water for 10–15 minutes. Then remove it from the heat and allow it to rest for five minutes. Finely chop your onion and garlic and fry them in a pan with a teaspoon of olive oil until they start to brown. Remove the pan from the heat. Chop up your tomato and roughly tear up your basil leaves. Combine your tomato, basil, garlic and onion with your quinoa, adding in a pinch of chilli flakes for an optional kick.

Halve your pepper and remove the seeds, then fill the halves with your quinoa mixture. Add the grated cheese on top and grill on a medium heat for 10–15 minutes. You can pack these up and eat them cold, or use your microwave at work to heat them up. If you have access to a cooker, you can pre-prepare these in the morning and grill them right before eating.

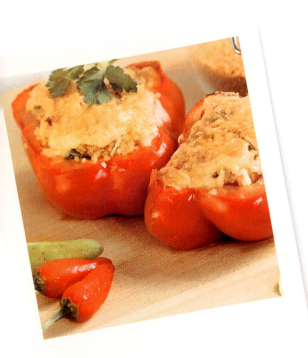

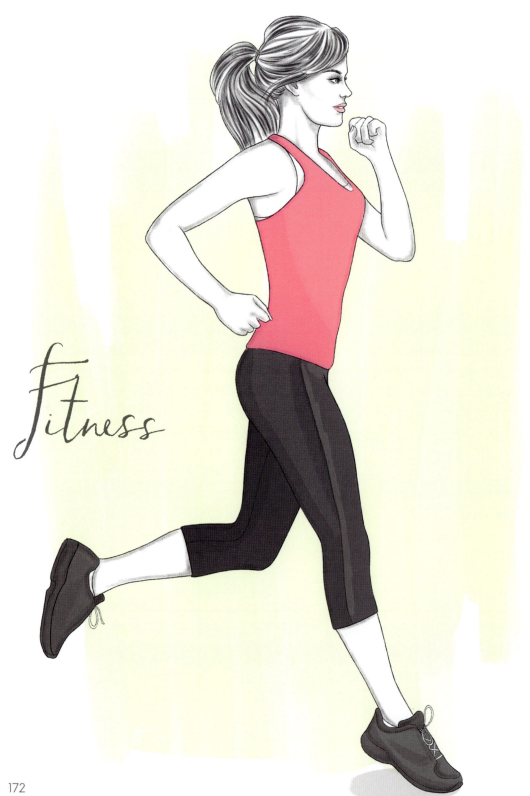

Fitness

When it comes to fitness and working out, it's all about discovering what works for you. Everyone has a different preference for what they like to do to keep fit, and how often they do it. As a rule, I try to get active three times a week. Whether it's going to the gym, taking a class or just going on a really long walk with my dogs, mixing it up helps me to stay interested and motivated, as I'm not a natural fitness fanatic. I always feel envious of those people who don't have to work hard to keep interested. If you struggle to keep yourself motivated, or frequently get stuck in a bit of a fitness rut, then I hope my advice helps you out!

FITNESS MATHS

Something I like to do every now and again to keep me motivated to stay fit and healthy is 'fitness maths'. Working out how much exercise you would have to do to burn off your favourite junk food is a great way to motivate yourself to eat more healthily and keep your cravings at bay. It's also quite fun too! Here are some of my favourite workout vs. junk food calculations. Obviously these are all based on averages, and the exact maths will depend on your weight, sex and speed, but it's a good way to put junk food into perspective!

1 Glazed Donut = 200 calories = 1 hour of cleaning the house

1 bar of Milk Chocolate = 250 calories = 1 hour of walking at a moderate speed

1 Slice of Takeaway Pizza = 250 calories = 30 minutes swimming at a moderate pace.

½ Tub of Ice Cream = 600 calories = Running 6 miles in 1 hour

Burger & Chips = 860 calories = 2 hours of rowing at a moderate speed

Fitness Shortcuts

If you're going to take the time and effort to get into the gym on a regular basis, you want to make sure that you are getting the most out of your workout every time. Here are my tips for making the most of your time in the gym, and maximising the results you get in return.

It's Not Always About Time

Well-planned 30-40 minute workouts can be more effective than spending hours in the gym training inefficiently. Plan out your workout to ensure you're making the most of every minute.

Mix It Up

If you stick to the same exercise routine every time you work out, your body will get used to it and the effectiveness will be reduced. Change up your workout every time, or alternate your workouts, so you continue to see the benefits in the long term.

Don't Rest During Your Workout

Instead of resting in between reps, move on to work on another part of your body. Circuit training in this way will make the most of your time in the gym and ensure you see results more quickly.

Perfect Your Form

Having the best possible posture and form during your workout will ensure you get the most out of your exercises. Poor form can sometimes cause damage, so make sure you keep your posture aligned and core engaged during your exercise.

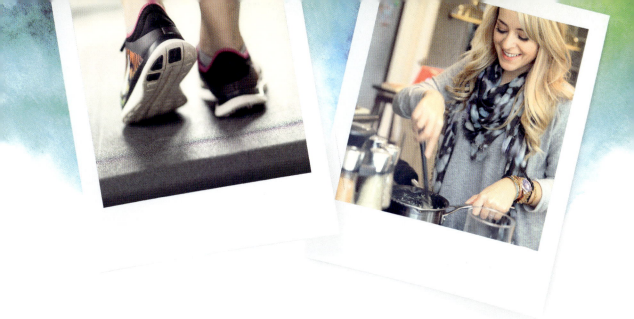

Find a Workout Buddy

Having someone to work out with not only gives a reason not to cancel your workout when you are feeling less than motivated, but it also adds an element of competition. A little bit of healthy competition is a great thing when it comes to working out, as it helps you to push yourself further and not give up when you get tired.

Pack in the Protein

Eating protein after your workout can help you to see results more quickly, as it both repairs and builds muscle, whether it's a protein shake or simply a boiled egg for a post-workout breakfast. Just be sure you aren't getting more than you need. Pay attention to labels and work out exactly how much protein you should be consuming for your sex, size and fitness.

Hydration

Keep hydrated by drinking water before, during and after exercise. Water reduces recovery time and fatigue, making for a more efficient workout.

Be Careful with Carbs

Avoiding carbs entirely has become something of a trend in recent years, but it's a misconception that totally excluding carbs is healthy. Carbohydrates are an essential part of your diet, and if you're going to exercise on a regular basis, you will need them for energy. Avoid simple carbs (such as refined sugar) when you can, and instead opt for complex carbs which are made up of longer chains of sugar molecules and take longer for the body to break down and turn into energy. These include legumes such as beans, pulses such as lentils, and whole grains such as quinoa.

Keeping Motivated

Keeping motivated is the hardest part of sticking to a healthy-eating and exercise routine. Doing nothing is always the easiest option, so how do you keep motivated to get off the sofa and into the gym?

Inspiration

Looking to those who have achieved and maintained a level of fitness or a lifestyle that you aspire to is a great way to keep motivated. However, you also need to bear in mind that everyone is different, and the way someone else looks is not always an achievable aspiration.

Positive Thinking

If you don't think positively, sticking to a routine and motivating yourself to keep fit and healthy will be nearly impossible. Whenever you start to lose your positive outlook on being healthy, take a step back and try to think about why you wanted to be healthy in the first place. Looking at the big picture when it comes to health is one of the easiest ways to remain positive and resist the temptation to break your routine.

Put It Down on Paper

Write down your goals and fitness aspirations and pin them to your fridge or wall. This will help you stick to them, as you'll be reminded of them on a daily basis.

Reward Yourself

Whether it's an experience, piece of clothing or new trainers, reward yourself each time you reach one of your personal goals. This will encourage you to keep striving to achieve your goals over a longer period of time.

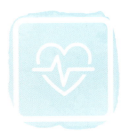

Take a Day Off

It's important to incorporate 'cheat days', or days off, into your routine to keep yourself motivated. Cheat days not only satisfy your cravings for food that you may be restricting the rest of the time, but they also provide something to look forward to in your routine.

Keep Track of Your Progress

Keeping track of your progress is the best way to keep motivated, as you'll be able to see how far you've come. It will enable you to set more realistic goals and monitor your progress towards achieving them.

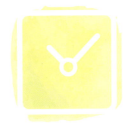

Use Technology to Your Advantage

There are so many apps available for tracking your nutrition and fitness. I find these one of the best ways to stick to a routine. My favourite apps are My Fitness Pal and My Diet Diary. Fitness wristbands are also a great way of tracking your progress and keeping yourself motivated, although they are a lot more expensive than an app.

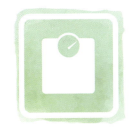

Get Your Gear On!

I feel twice as motivated to work out if I'm wearing gym gear. You'll be less likely to make an excuse or change your mind when it comes to getting into the gym.

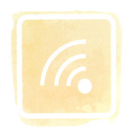

10 Quick Tips

Don't Cut Out Fat

You're right in thinking that saturated fat is bad for you, but good fat is essential for your health. Integrate it into your diet by eating foods such as avocado, nuts and coconut oil.

Think of What You Could Do in Half an Hour

You can easily lose 30 minutes mindlessly browsing the internet. Think about how else you could spend your time. That 30 minutes would be much more beneficial spent in the gym, or going for a walk or a quick run outside.

If Something in Your Routine Isn't Working, Change It!

There's no point forcing yourself to do something that doesn't work for you. Find something that does work for you and do that instead. Otherwise you'll risk giving up entirely.

'I Don't Have the Energy' Isn't an Excuse

Moderate exercise has been proven to actually give you more energy, so don't use fatigue as an excuse to avoid working out. It'll make you feel better in the long run.

Exhale on the Effort

Breathing out as you exert effort will help you tone up more quickly, making the most of your exercises.

Make a Playlist

It sounds obvious, but making a playlist before you hit the gym or head out for a run will help to keep you motivated during your workout, and save you fiddling with your phone to find a good song.

Work Out First Thing

Working out in the morning before you eat means you won't just be burning off your breakfast. Follow an early morning workout with a protein-rich breakfast.

Boost Your Mood

Eating food rich in certain vitamins and minerals (including vitamin B and omega-3 fatty acids) has been proven to boost your mood. Try eating dark chocolate (with over 70 per cent cocoa solids), salmon or dark vegetables such as broccoli and peppers for their natural mood-enhancing properties.

Time Your Sugar Right

Treating yourself to dessert every now and again is not a bad thing, but timing your sweet treats right can help to minimise the effects of sugar on your body. If you can, wait two hours after your meal to eat dessert, as the sugar can impede the absorption of nutrients.

Sleep Is All Important

Getting enough sleep is essential for all aspects of your health. Depriving your body of sleep can not only accelerate the ageing process, but being tired can also have an impact on your motivation for a healthy lifestyle. Nothing pushes you to reach for the junk food more than a lack of sleep!

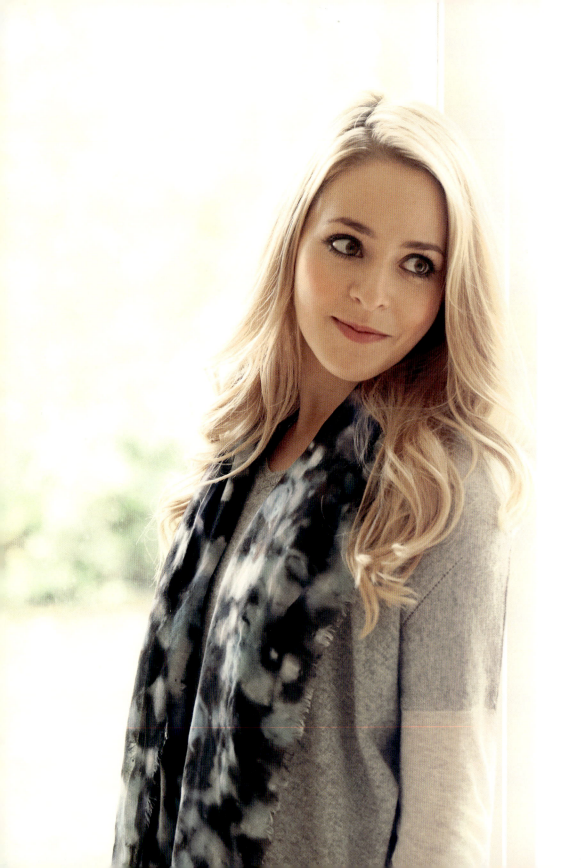

Life, Love,

Dreams and

Everything In Between

Introduction

This chapter is something of a departure from the topics I've covered in this book so far. When I asked my online audience what they would like to see in a book from me, there was a flood of requests for tips on improving self-confidence and body image, so I knew it was something I couldn't omit from the contents. Women have never been under as much pressure as they are today. Whether it's the expectation to look a certain way, have the perfect work–life balance or maintain a 'perfect' relationship, these pressures understandably affect most women's state of mind. It's important to take a step back from normal life every now and then to assess how this pressure is affecting your outlook and your own personal happiness and development.

This chapter will not only cover the issues of self-confidence and body image, but will also offer advice for learning to think more positively about your life as a whole. I've also included tips for reading your dreams, to enable you to better understand issues and insecurities clear only to your subconscious, and advice for dating and relationships, to help you navigate the world of love a little easier.

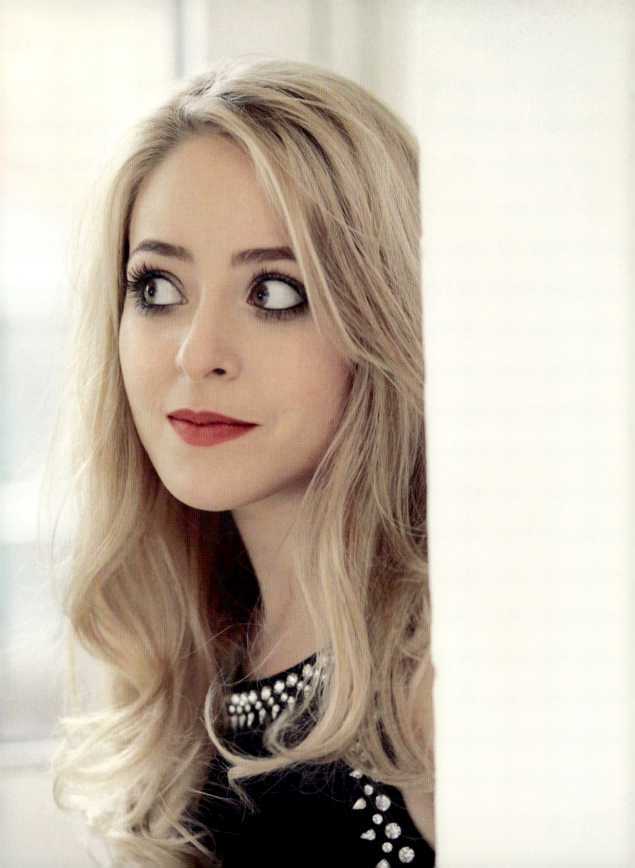

Self-Confidence

Having been bullied in my younger years, a lack of self-confidence held me back for a long time. A fear of failure often stopped me from following my dreams and trying new things, but after years of battling with confidence issues, I've finally learnt how to get the better of them and be more sure of myself and my ability to succeed.

Self-confidence relates to your self-assurance in your personal judgement and ability to succeed in life. A lack of self-confidence leads to you to have an unnecessary reliance on the approval and opinions of others. Some people may have confidence in some areas of their life, but not in others, so it's all about isolating which areas you need to work on. Positive yet realistic is the ideal (being over-confident is never a good thing), but it can be hard to strike the right balance.

Before you can take action, you need to take a step back and look at where you are now, what your strengths and weaknesses are and where you feel you're lacking belief in yourself. Once you've identified what aspects could do with some work, bear in mind the following advice and tips for improving your self-confidence in practical situations.

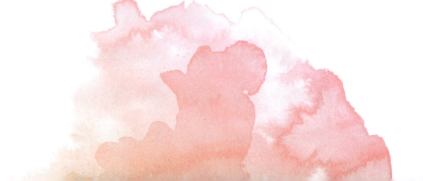

YOU DON'T HAVE TO CONFORM IN ORDER TO BE ACCEPTED

Being like everyone else is often the easier thing to do in life, but it doesn't make you happier in the long run. Learning to love who you are and allowing yourself to do what makes you happy regardless of what other people think is the key to being happy and confident in your life choices.

TAKE RISKS

Taking risks can be scary, but it is the only way to push yourself into trying new things. Make yourself step out of your comfort zone. Even if you don't achieve what you initially set out to do, the process itself is a confidence-building experience.

ACKNOWLEDGE THE EFFORT YOU MAKE RATHER THAN THE END RESULT

People with low self-confidence often concentrate only on their failings, or the end result of a process. If you give yourself credit for the effort and progress you've made, you're likely to feel more confident in yourself, knowing that you've tried and achieved something rather than criticising yourself for not fulfilling your initial expectations.

FOCUS ON YOUR STRENGTHS AND TALENTS, AND BUILD ON THEM IF YOU NEED TO

Everyone has their weaknesses, therefore everyone lacks confidence in certain areas. Focus on where your strengths lie and remember them at times when you're feeling negative. Also remember that a little hard work can turn weaknesses into strengths. Studying or practising in areas you don't feel confident or knowledgeable in will not only help in a practical way, but it will boost your all-round self-confidence too.

LEARN TO ACCEPT COMPLIMENTS GRACEFULLY

Nothing highlights a lack of self-confidence more than rejecting or reacting awkwardly to praise and admiration. Once you learn to accept compliments with a smile and thanks, you'll start to believe them and let them make you feel good about yourself.

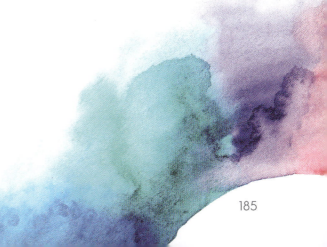

PRACTICAL STEPS

It's all very well striving to improve your self-confidence in theory, but what about when you're not feeling as confident as you would like in a situation and you need an immediate solution to give you a confidence boost, or to fake the appearance of it at least!

Adopt a Confident Pose

It's been scientifically proven that your body language has a direct effect on your mental state. Adopting a 'strong' pose will help to temporarily improve your self-confidence. Straighten your posture, put your hands on your hips and raise your head high. Slouching or holding your arms across your body in a protective stance are weak poses and should be avoided when you're feeling nervous, as these gestures can exacerbate feelings of anxiety and nervousness.

Dress for the Occasion

Dressing well is a great way to give yourself an instant confidence boost. Wearing high heels can help improve your posture and also give you extra height, which can have a similar effect.

Smile

Smiling is a great way to fake confidence: not only do you fool those around you, you can also trick yourself into feeling more assured. Crack a smile when you feel nervous. It will make you feel better and those around you will assume you're totally unfazed by the situation at hand.

Speak Up

Speaking quietly, mumbling or struggling with words is an instant giveaway if you're feeling shy. Try your best to speak loudly and clearly, as this is another sign of being confident and self-assured. Keep an even, clear tone when talking to people. This will mask insecurities and also save you the embarrassment of having to repeat yourself when you're already feeling nervous.

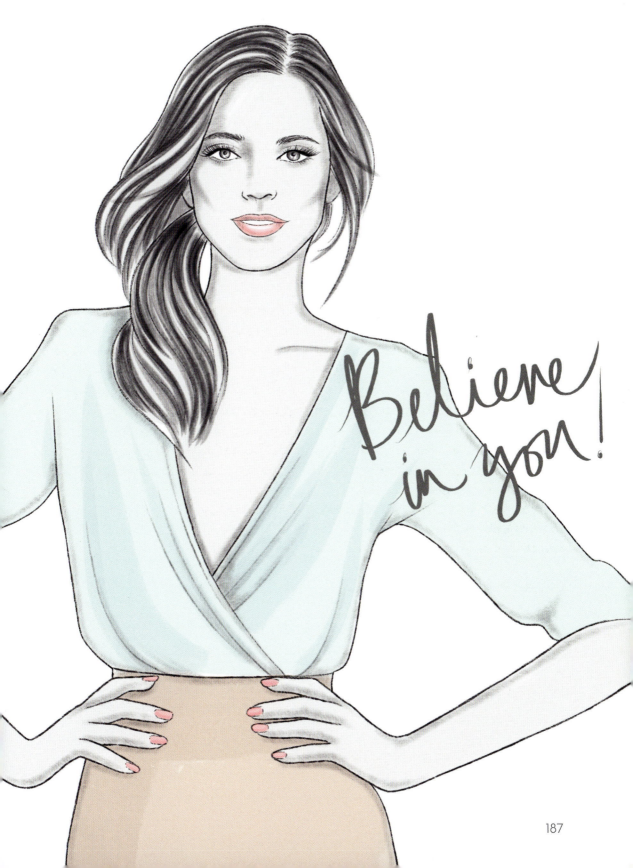

Believe in you!

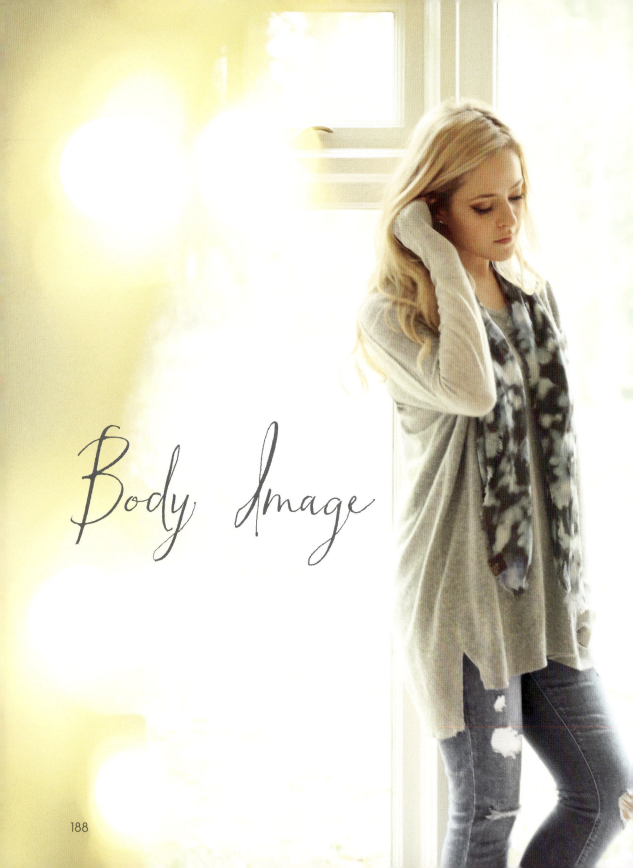

Body Image

Although body image is intrinsically linked to self-confidence and positive thinking, I thought it deserved a section of its own in this book, as there has never been more pressure on young girls and women to look a certain way than there is today. There are very few women I know who truly love their body. It's something that most of us struggle with on a daily basis. However, once you learn to think positively about your figure and start loving your body, it will make you so much happier. Negative body image is something that has affected every woman at some point in her life, and a lot of the blame has to be pointed at the media feeding us unattainable images of what is perceived to be the 'ideal' female body. Here are my tips for fighting back against this constant pressure and taking steps towards learning to truly love your figure.

STOP COMPARING YOURSELF TO OTHERS

This is the number one most important step when it comes to having a positive, healthy relationship with your body. Everyone is different, and every single person has a feature they don't like. Most of the time other people notice only the best assets in others and the worst in themselves, so comparing yourself to others is never a constructive way to think.

IDENTIFY YOUR BEST ASSETS AND FOCUS ON THEM

Once you've identified what you love about the way you look, you can start building a positive body image from there. Start by making a list of all the things that you like about yourself. When you are getting dressed or getting ready in the mornings, draw attention to these features with the help of your clothes and makeup. Highlighting your assets will make you feel more confident in yourself and happy in your own skin.

STOP CRITICISING OTHER WOMEN

The move towards positive body image in society as a whole is not going to be an easy one, but if it is going to happen, women need to stop criticising other women's bodies. Highlighting someone else's imperfections isn't going to improve the way you think about yourself, and will only feed your own insecurity.

ADMIRE SUCCESSFUL WOMEN

Admiration based on appearance won't help you to conquer body-image problems or provide you with worthwhile role models. Once you start to admire women for the right reasons (actual achievement), you'll start to be able to put things into perspective a little more and realise that appearance isn't the be all and end all.

TAKE A CLOSER LOOK AT NATURE

Nothing in the natural world is perfect in the way an airbrushed photograph is. Take a look outside and you'll see that the natural world is full of beautiful imperfections. The idolisation of the perfect appearance is a man-made obsession; the beauty of the natural world is that everything is different and imperfect in its own way.

FIND ONE THING TO COMPLIMENT YOURSELF ON EACH DAY

Whether it's clear skin, a good hair day, or seeing the results of last week's workout on a particular part of your body, don't forget to appreciate the parts of your body that you like and that you're proud of.

WEAR CLOTHING THAT MAKES YOU FEEL GOOD

When you're unhappy with the way you look, it's tempting to wear loose-fitting clothing to cover up, but in reality this only lowers your body confidence and makes you feel worse about your figure. Choose clothes that make you feel your best for an instant body-confidence boost.

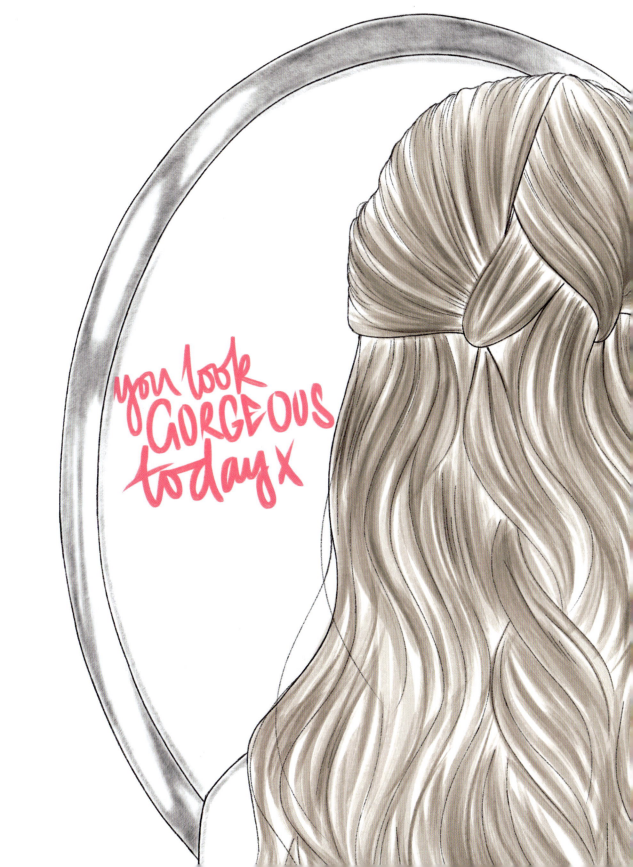

Positive Thinking

Positive thinking doesn't just make you happier, it actually has proven health benefits too. It's been scientifically proven to reduce stress, which can lead to a longer life span and a reduced risk of cardiovascular disease and depression in the long run. If you're not naturally a positive thinker, it can be hard to train your brain to be optimistic all of the time, but the following tips have really helped me to become more positive and to deal with stress and negativity over the past few years.

TURN YOUR THOUGHTS AROUND

It's almost impossible to stop thinking negative thoughts entirely, but you can make a pact with yourself to turn them into positive ones. As soon as you notice you are starting to think negatively, try to stamp out that thought and replace it with a positive one.

SURROUND YOURSELF WITH POSITIVE PEOPLE

Both positive and negative thinking are contagious. If you surround yourself with happy people, you're likely to be happier yourself. It's also worth thinking about limiting the time you spend with negative people, or those who bring you down, as they will have the opposite effect.

REMEMBER THAT
NO ONE IS PERFECT

Lingering on negative experiences or actions won't help you or anyone else in your life. Learn from your mistakes and move on; don't dwell on them with negative feelings.

MAKE A LIST OF ALL THE THINGS YOU ARE THANKFUL FOR IN YOUR LIFE

This is a great way to realise how much you have to be positive about, as the list is usually longer than you'd think!

KEEP WORKING ON IT

Positive thinking isn't something you can simply turn on and off. You have to keep working on it as you go through life. If you are a natural pessimist, positive thinking can take a lot of work and the tips above take a lot of practice before they become second nature. Over time it will become easier and easier.

DON'T BE AFRAID TO ASK FOR HELP

Asking your friends and family for help or extra support when you need it is one of the best ways to stay positive when you are struggling. Let those closest to you know what you're trying to achieve and ask them to help you stick to it. They'll often be the first to see you slipping back into negative thought patterns.

First Date Etiquette

First dates are, without a doubt, one of the most nerve-wracking social encounters you will experience. Awkward moments are inevitable, but the potential to find love is undeniably exciting and there's no other social encounter like it. Here are my tips for making the first date itself less awkward and intimidating, so you can concentrate on charming your date!

CHOOSING THE RIGHT VENUE

If you are the one choosing the venue, take a little time to think about where you want to go. You don't want to pick somewhere too pricey or formal, as that can not only give off the wrong impression about expecting your date to foot the bill, but it also sets the tone for the evening. Think casual and mid-price range but still romantic.

TIME YOUR ARRIVAL

There is nothing worse than being stood up. However, this is also true for the guy! When it comes to timings, try to be almost on time. I think being five minutes late is optimal. In an ideal scenario you want to arrive after him, to avoid appearing overly keen, but any later than that and you risk being a little rude!

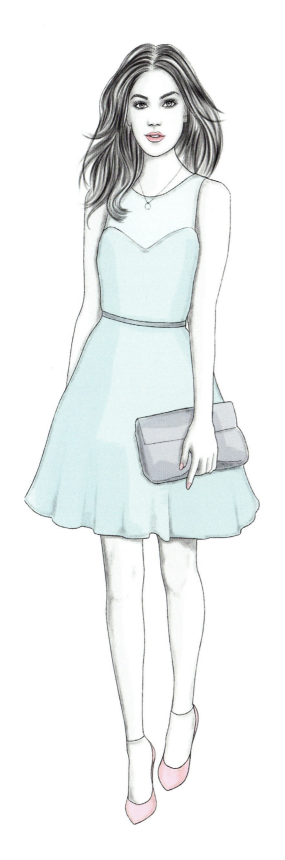

THE OUTFIT

You want to keep it casual and perhaps a bit flirty. Avoid anything too short or low cut, but keep a little something intriguing about your outfit. A pretty dress and nice heels is a good choice, depending on the venue. Most importantly, wear something you feel comfortable and confident in. If you feel uncomfortable, you'll look uncomfortable. Stick to what you know you look your best in.

CONVERSATION

Try to keep the conversation balanced. Ask him questions whenever appropriate. The first date is a great opportunity to find out all about someone, but remember not to dig too deeply and avoid talking about controversial subjects like religion, ex-partners, money and politics. Save serious topics for the second date! Keeping the conversation light-hearted and fun is the best way to avoid any potential awkwardness. It's also essential to keep your phone in your bag and on silent throughout the date. Nothing else spoils an atmosphere like your phone going off during a meal, or constantly checking your emails during a conversation. Keep your phone hidden and your eyes on your date at all times!

WHAT TO EAT

People always recommend avoiding difficult-to-eat dishes on first dates, which is true to a certain extent, but if a guy is put off by you struggling over spaghetti, then that's probably a sign he's not 'The One' anyway! Order what you want, but it's best practice not to order the most expensive thing on the menu, as this can give off the impression that you're expecting him to pay. It's also best to go easy on the garlic in case the date goes exceptionally well! When you're eating, remember to take small mouthfuls. If the conversation is flowing, you don't want to create an awkward silence while you chew on a huge chunk of steak, or risk talking with your mouth full. Also be careful not to drink too much! One or two drinks are more than enough to calm your nerves and ease conversation. Getting drunk on a first date is a huge no-no.

FOOTING THE BILL

When it comes to paying the bill, most gentlemen offer to take care of it, but it's important to offer to split the bill before he's had a chance to pay. When the bill comes, reach for your purse and politely offer to pay. If he declines, don't argue too much (being too pushy can be downright annoying and some guys take it quite personally if the girl doesn't let them pay). If you end up splitting the bill, don't be offended. It's traditional for the guy to pay, but it's also an acknowledgement of you being on equal terms if he lets you cover your half of the bill.

THE GOODBYE

The end of the night has the potential to be either the most awkward moment or the highlight of the evening. If the date goes badly and you never want to see him again, give him a hug or handshake, say, 'Nice to meet you,' and leave it at that! If it goes well, give him a hug and a kiss on the cheek, but wait for him to make the plans for a second date. If it goes really well, a goodnight kiss is appropriate, but always leave it at that on the first date.

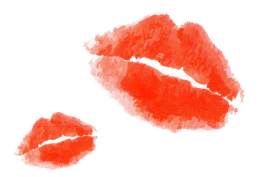

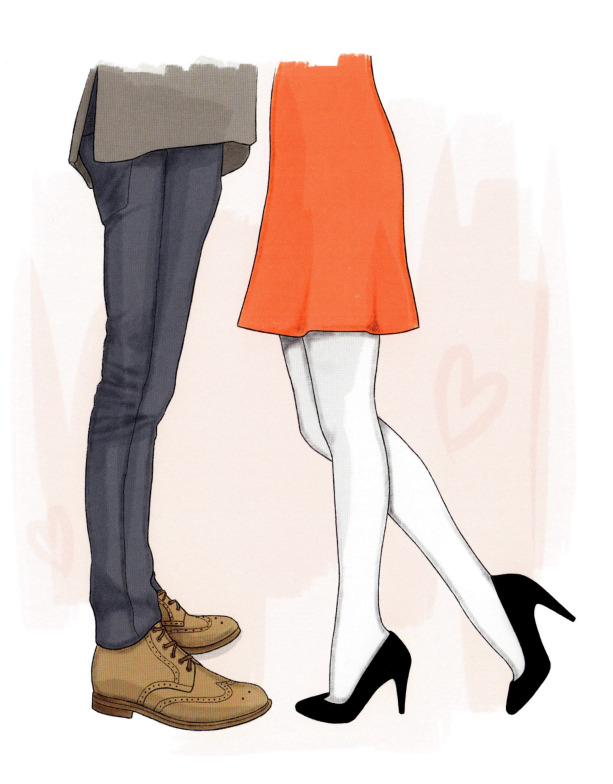

Making Relationships Last

There is no magical secret to making a relationship last. Working out how to balance your lives in harmony with each other and learning how to make the most of what each of you bring to the relationship is a tricky endeavour. Long-term relationships are never going to be all roses. Every couple goes through rough patches and blissful periods, but you can make the journey smoother by investing a little time and effort into your relationship when and where you need to. Here are my tips for making your relationship stand the test of time.

SPEAK UP ABOUT HOW YOU FEEL

Not letting your partner know how you're feeling is counter-productive and will only serve to exacerbate the problem.

COMPROMISE

Even if you have quite a stubborn personality (like me!) it's important to learn how to compromise in any relationship. You can't always be right or have things go your way. The basis of a successful relationship is finding a compromise between what you both want. Of course, some of the time you'll want to argue it out, but sometimes you have to agree to disagree and find a middle ground.

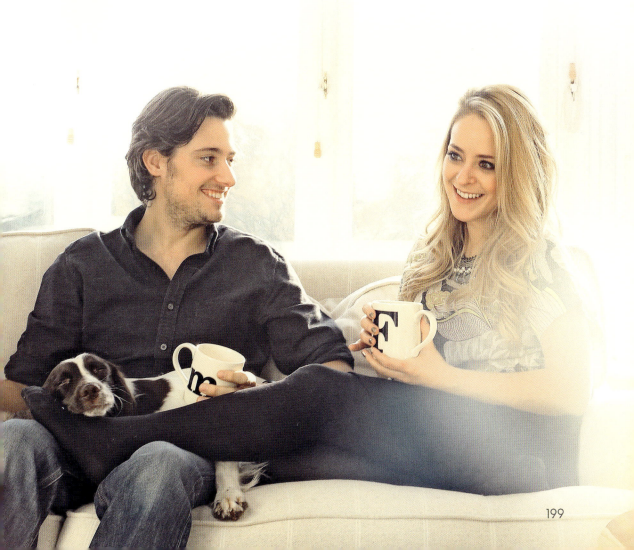

LEARN TO SAY YOU'RE SORRY, AND MEAN IT

Even if it's a case of swallowing your pride, learning to apologise is something you have to do in any long-term relationship.

LEARN TO LISTEN TO EACH OTHER

If you have a problem, argument or difference of opinion, it's important to listen to each other's reasoning and change your outlook accordingly.

BE HONEST WITH EACH OTHER

This is, above anything else, the foundation for a successful relationship. Being open with each other about how you feel is essential. As soon as you start holding things back, or telling white lies, you're letting cracks work their way into your relationship and they can be hard to patch up.

MAKE TIME FOR ROMANCE

It's easy to get carried away with work, socialising and life in general, but it's so important to make time for romance in any relationship. No matter how long you've been together, planning date nights or romantic getaways is something you should factor into your lives on a regular basis. Great relationships take work, so don't let yourself neglect something that's taken years to build.

HAVE FUN

As with making time for each other, it's easy for life to get in the way of having fun. Take the time to enjoy each other's company and have fun together.

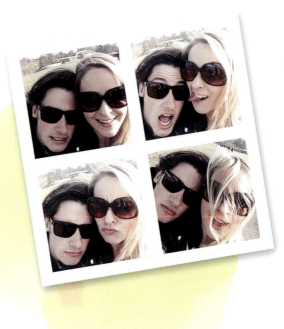

REMIND YOURSELF WHY YOU LOVE THEM

In times of doubt, or after an argument, make a mental list of all the things you love about your partner. This is a great way to put things into perspective and remind yourself why you got together in the first place, and why it's worth working on your relationship to make it last.

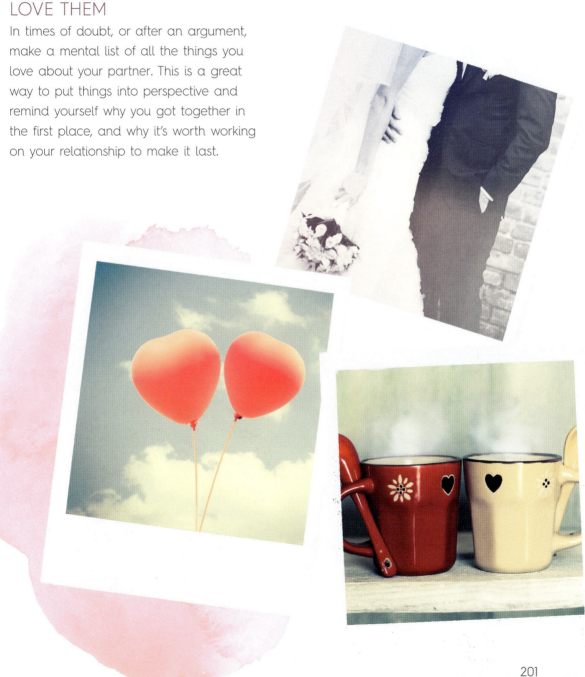

Life Goals

They may be short-term goals for the next six months or life-long aspirations, but setting goals in your life is one of the best ways to help you realise your dreams and get to where you want to be. It's easy to get swept up in your daily life and lose sight of the big picture. The fast pace of the modern world often leaves us with little time to take a step back and think about where our lives are taking us, but if you put a little effort into envisioning goals, it really can help you take a new direction.

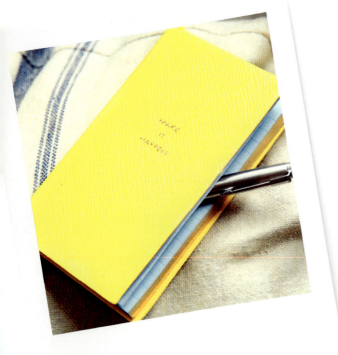

STEP 1

Take a step back and think about what you want to achieve within a set period of time. These goals can be as loose or as specific as you like. It's very important to make sure you can track your progress, so that you can work out a realistic schedule for yourself. Your aims have to be genuinely attainable. You want your goals to push you to a certain extent, but setting impossible ones which you know you will never achieve is counter-productive and will not leave you feeling satisfied or happy as an end result.

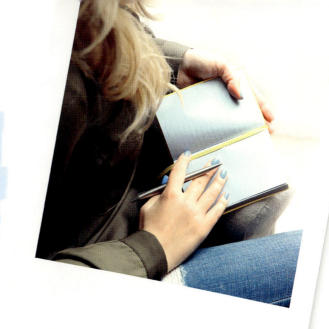

STEP 2

Break these larger aspirations down into individual achievements (for example, if you want to run a marathon in six months' time, you might want to set bi-weekly distance targets). This works for pretty much any aspect of your life, from fitness to financial, career, educational and relationship aspirations. If your goal is lifelong, try setting a five-year plan, one-year plan, six-month plan and one-month plan. Once you achieve your first goal, you can go on to set another. It's all about breaking down something that seems daunting and unattainable into smaller, manageable achievements over shorter periods of time. By doing this, you can not only see progress being made more quickly, but you will also stay motivated.

STEP 3

Get to work. Now they're broken down, your goals seem much less daunting.

STEP 4

Review and update your progress on a regular basis. Whether it's amending your aims constantly as you go along or stopping every few months to reassess your situation, keep tweaking them over time to keep them relevant and you'll have a clearer vision in your head of the end result.

Reading Your Dreams

The average person spends one third of their life sleeping and six years (or about 2,100 whole days) dreaming. In an average night you are likely to dream for about one or two hours, but it's not uncommon to dream for longer than that. Even if you don't remember anything about your dreams, that doesn't mean you're not having them. Everyone dreams, without exception, and your dreams serve as a window to your subconscious, giving you an insight into how you perceive yourself. They are, however, often incredibly difficult to remember beyond the first few moments after waking. Remembering your dreams allows you to gain knowledge about your subconscious and increase your self-awareness, and helps you to tackle any psychological issues you may have, no matter how big or small.

Keeping track of your dreams and deciphering their meaning is a great way to facilitate self-healing and help to conquer any social or emotional issues you are suffering from. Here is a quick summary of some common dream scenarios and an insight into what they can mean. If you're interested in exploring the world of dreams in more depth, I'd recommend investing in a dictionary of dreams.

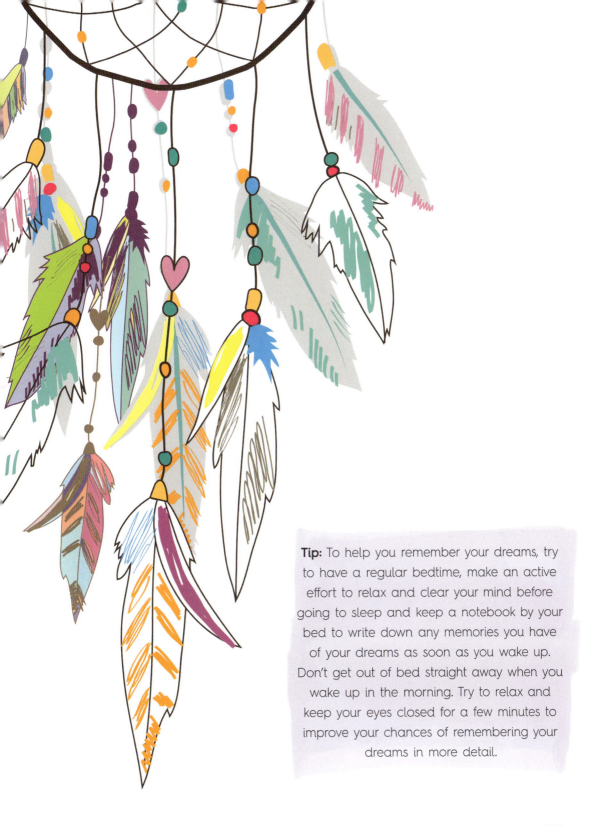

Tip: To help you remember your dreams, try to have a regular bedtime, make an active effort to relax and clear your mind before going to sleep and keep a notebook by your bed to write down any memories you have of your dreams as soon as you wake up. Don't get out of bed straight away when you wake up in the morning. Try to relax and keep your eyes closed for a few minutes to improve your chances of remembering your dreams in more detail.

Death dreams have a variety of different influences and potential meanings. A lot of the time they signify a change in your life. Pay attention to who or what is dying in your dream, as it often signifies the loss of something associated with that person. Death dreams can actually be quite positive, and signify the need to move on from certain issues or influences in your life. Most importantly, don't take death dreams too literally, or associate them with a bad omen.

Being chased in your dreams can signify anxiety in your life. It's important to focus on who is chasing you and why. Chasing dreams are often linked to avoidance, fear of something, or self-denial (the latter especially so if you are running away from yourself).

Falling dreams are usually closely linked to a current situation or feeling in your life, rather than something more deeply rooted. It might be an insecurity or a loss of control. Don't be surprised or worried by falling dreams if you are going through a stressful time in your life, as they can often be directly attributed to feelings of instability and a lack of confidence.

Flying dreams are often amongst the best dreams and are usually positive experiences. Flying above things can signify moving on or getting over obstacles in your life and achieving freedom from things that hold you back. I often have dreams about struggling to get off the ground, managing to fly for a few metres but coming quickly back down to the ground. While this is a fairly common occurrence in dreams, it can be frustrating and tends to signify a lack of confidence or motivation.

Exam dreams are another of the most common and can often occur when you have no upcoming actual test in your life. They usually signify nervousness, a fear of failure or a lack of confidence for an upcoming challenge, whatever form it may take. The main focus during exam or test dreams should be the *process* rather than the content of the test itself. Try to focus on the experience of being tested, rather than what's in the test in order to pinpoint the source of the issue.

Cheating dreams are very common and usually stem from low self-esteem or trust issues within your relationship. Try to identify why you might feel at risk from your partner cheating. Often it might be due to lack of attention or other issues in your relationship, but a lot of the time it stems from simple insecurity.

Naked dreams often represent insecurity, fear of exposure, vulnerability, falling short of your goals or being unprepared for a task at hand.

Teeth dreams are also fairly common. Dreams in which you are losing your teeth often signify an underlying insecurity about your looks or fears of public embarrassment, but also communication problems or feelings of powerlessness or concern over health issues.

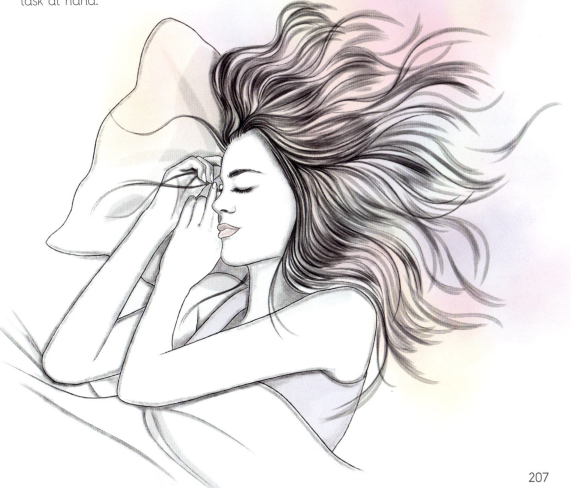

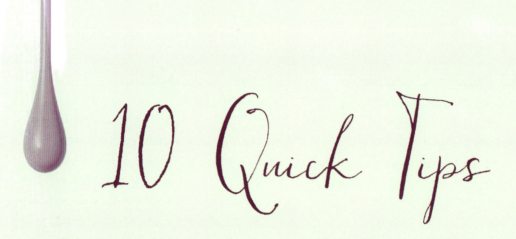

10 Quick Tips

Focus on the Present Moment

It's the only place where you can physically be and have total control over. It's all very well planning for the future or dwelling on the past, but if you neglect the present, you won't enjoy the journey.

Take Time Out

If you're feeling stressed or pressured about any aspect of your life, it's really important to take some time out for yourself and allow yourself to reassess the situation or problem.

Learn from Past Experience

It might seem like obvious advice, but looking back and learning from negative experiences in the past will help you to avoid the same outcome in the future and allow you to move on.

Find Something to Laugh About

Laughter is one of the easiest ways to make yourself feel better, no matter what you're going through. If you ever need a quick emotional pick-me-up, think back to a moment in your life that makes you laugh.

See Each Day as a Challenge

When your life seems overwhelmingly busy, see each day as a challenge. If you wake up motivated and go to sleep satisfied at having achieved your daily goal, it makes the big picture look a lot more manageable.

Don't Expect Change to Be Easy

Whether it's in your thinking, lifestyle or relationship, never expect a big change in your life to be easy. Most changes take time, work and emotional adjustment. Seeing change as a real challenge will help you to stay motivated and to keep your outlook positive.

Remember that Your Present Situation Is Temporary

No matter what negative space you're in, it's only temporary. You can change any aspect of your life if you work hard enough.

Look at Your Life in a Different Light

Once you start thinking about something in a certain way, it's hard to get away from that way of thinking. If you have a pressure or obstacle in your life that you are struggling to overcome, take a look at it from a different angle, or try to identify what you're *not* currently seeing, as this can be the key to conquering the problem in the long run.

Start Small

You can't expect to change the way you think about life, yourself or a relationship overnight. Start with small adaptations that can develop into big changes over time.

Don't Put Off Change

If there's something you want to change about your life, start now. It's so easy to make excuses, but there is no time like the present!

YouTube and Blogging

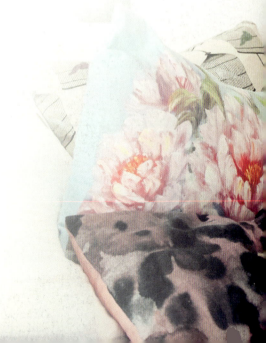

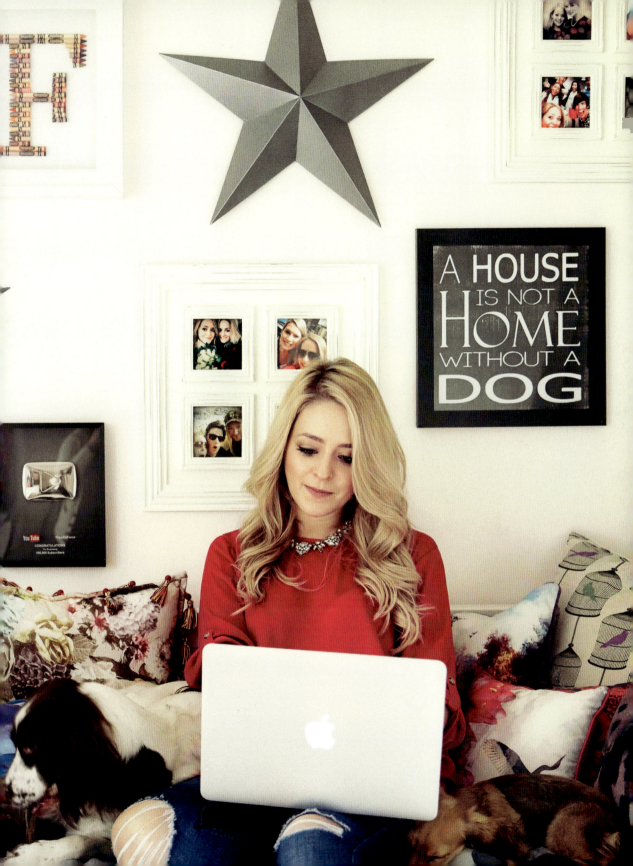

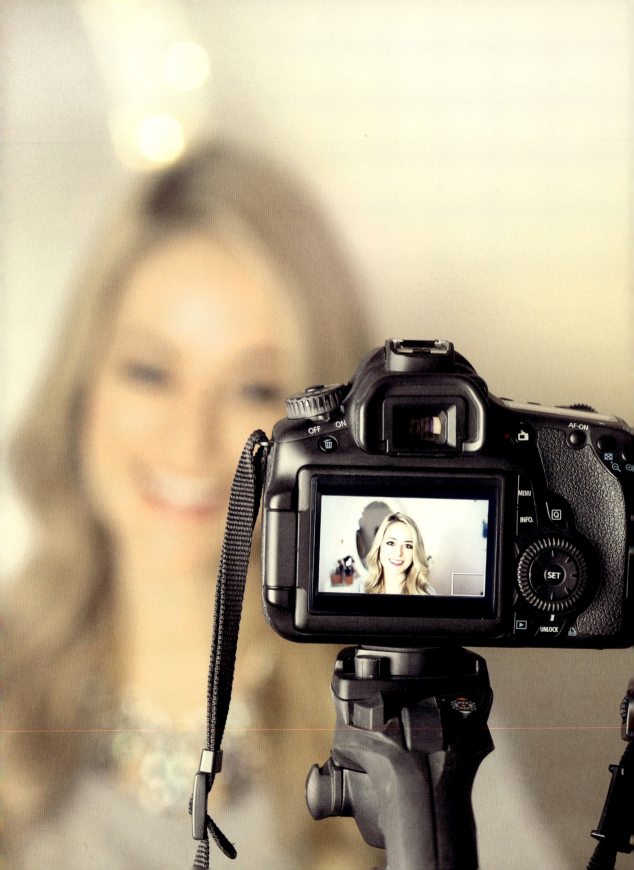

Introduction

So many people ask me for advice when it comes to starting a YouTube channel. Whether it's the equipment you need, how to talk to the camera, how to make your channel unique, or how to deal with haters, there is always a preconception that starting to make videos on YouTube requires some kind of skill base, investment or specialised knowledge. That is totally unfounded. The beautiful thing about YouTube is that anyone can start a channel, on any budget. As long as you have a camera of some kind and a laptop on which to upload your videos, the world of YouTube is your oyster.

I strongly advise anyone thinking of starting a channel to simply *do it*. Try it out for yourself and see if you like it. If you do, and people start to watch, think about improving your production quality at that point. It's more about getting your content out there than how well it is shot and edited. If you are passionate about what you're talking about, that will come across naturally to the viewers. Another great thing about starting like this is that you learn as you go along. When I started making videos, I filmed them on my in-built webcam and learnt to use iMovie from scratch that day. My videos weren't perfect, but I learnt so much in the first couple of months. As I grew a small audience of viewers, they gave me amazing advice and suggestions on how to improve my content as I went along.

Because YouTube is so new and dynamic, it's constantly evolving and changing, and immersing yourself within the community really is the best way to truly understand what your audience wants, when they want it, and how to improve your content. Every channel is different, and will therefore have its own individual audience with different preferences and sensitivities, so it's more a case of getting to know *your own* community than the YouTube community as a whole.

With that in mind, here is some general advice I would give to anyone thinking about starting up a YouTube channel, or to those of you who have done so recently and want some tips on growing your audience. I hope this is useful, but please remember that there really is no better way to learn how to do something than by jumping in at the deep end and trying it out first-hand!

Equipment

WHAT CONTENT ARE YOU MAKING?

The kit you need is really determined by the type of content you make. If you are filming daily vlogs, for example, you don't need to worry about your camera being beautifully high quality and you don't need to worry about lighting too much, as it's more important that your kit is portable and simple to use. Think about exactly what kind of content you want to be making and what you need your equipment to be able to do.

CAMERAS

I find the best way to find out what I need is to ask. Go into a camera shop and ask their advice, or find a friend who knows a lot about cameras. Also remember that Google is your friend! There are so many tech reviews out there and reading lots of them is a sure-fire way to know if you're splashing your cash on the right camera.

What I Use

I use a Canon S120 for daily vlogging, and a Canon 60D with a Sigma 30mm lens for filming my beauty and fashion videos.

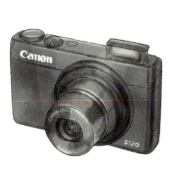 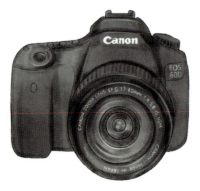 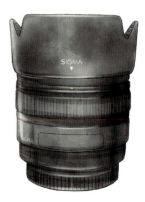

LIGHTING

Learning about basic lighting techniques will help a lot when it comes to setting up your videos. The most basic but useful approach for static YouTube videos is the 'three-point lighting' concept (see next page). There are a lot of tutorials on YouTube itself showing you how this works and how to apply it to a YouTube camera set-up, but it's essentially based on using three separate lighting sources to eliminate shadows on your subject. The main or 'key' light is placed directly facing your subject. The secondary or 'fill' light also shines on the subject, but from a side angle, slightly lower than the key light, to help illuminate any shadows, and the third 'back' light shines on the subject from behind, visually separating the subject from the background. There really is nothing better than natural lighting, so if you can shoot outside, do! Fashion videos always look better when shot outside.

What I Use

I use soft boxes to evenly diffuse the light in my videos, as they are affordable, collapsible and effective – you can buy them online for around £50 each. A ring light is also good to have when it comes to shooting beauty videos, as the 'ring' of light adds a touch of glamour to the overall footage by reducing shadows and lines on the face and adding a 'halo effect' to the eyes. They can be more expensive, but they're a good investment in the long run.

TRIPOD

There are so many different tripods available, but for YouTube it's often best to go for a travel option rather than a more sturdy one, as you might not always be filming in the same place. I travel a lot with my tripod, so it's useful to have one that collapses to a small size and is fairly lightweight.

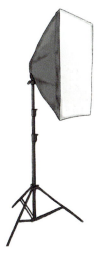
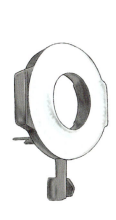
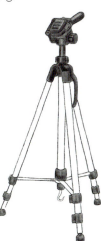

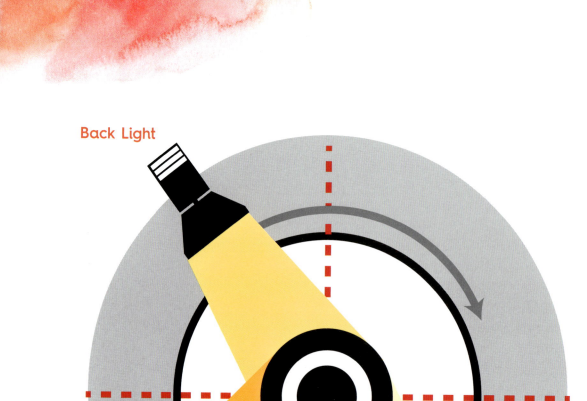

Back Light

Key Light

Fill Light

THREE-POINT LIGHTING GUIDE

Getting Inspired

The hardest part of making digital content, whether it's in written, video or photographic form, is getting inspiration. The nature of the internet means that you have to be consistently and frequently uploading new material in order to continue to grow and maintain an audience. Creativity isn't always a steady process, and inspiration is not always abundant. My ideas for new content come from three different sources in equal measure...

AUDIENCE FEEDBACK

My first and main source of concepts for new content is the instant response provided by my online audience. One of the most exciting elements of the digital space is that you can get immediate feedback on your work. If I do something a bit different and it proves to be popular, I can instantly take that on board and adapt future content to improve the audience's experience.

PERSONAL INTEREST

Expanding and improving your content based on your personal interests and passions as they change is also essential. I love trying out new ideas and video formats, and exploring topics I've recently become interested in. Although a lot of the time these may not be as popular as tried-and-tested formats, it's the best way to keep your material fresh and ensure that your content grows and develops with you over time.

OUTSIDE INSPIRATION

Whether it's a feature you've seen in a newspaper, a personal experience you've been through in your life, or a beautiful landscape you've encountered that day, sources of inspiration really are all around us. If I'm ever feeling stuck for ideas or feeling bored of the same production process, getting outside always helps. Whether you're in a bustling city or isolated countryside, exploring is a sure-fire source of inspiration.

Growing an Audience

One of the most common questions I get asked about YouTube and blogging is how to go about building your audience, and keeping that growth consistent. There are three simple tips I always give to ensure you are making the most of your potential to develop your own audience online, and to keep them interested in the long run:

Be Consistent. Set a schedule for your content and stick to it. This way your audience will know when to expect new content from you, and therefore when to come back to your site to look for updates. It also shows that you are worth the effort they make by incorporating your content into their daily, weekly or monthly routine.

Be Persistent. An audience doesn't simply appear overnight. It takes time and a huge amount of hard work and dedication to build and maintain a loyal audience. Be persistent and have patience.

Be Yourself. If you're in it for the long haul, you'll want to be true to yourself and your interests. Put across your real personality in your content. This way your audience is more likely to grow with you rather than grow out of you as both you and they change and develop. Trying to be something you're not gets old, quickly. Be yourself, and be as open as possible with your followers in order to make a deeper connection with them.

Tip: Don't let criticism get you down. Take criticism on board and move on. If it's constructive, let it serve as a means of highlighting any weakness in your current content. If it's mindless hate, don't engage with it and don't let it affect you. There are a lot of wonderful things about the internet, but trolls aren't one of them. Giving them attention only fuels their desire to upset you.

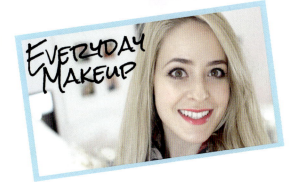

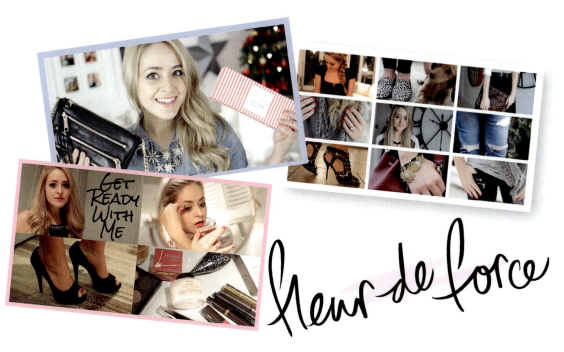

fleur de force

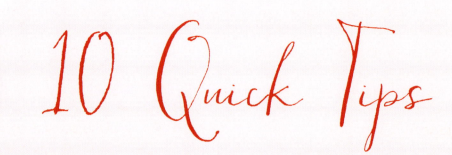

10 Quick Tips

Don't Forget Why You Started

Remembering why you fell in love with creating content in the first place is the key to staying motivated, inspired and true to yourself.

Don't Let Negativity Get in Your Way

The internet can breed negativity, but it's important to focus on the positive feedback and comments and never let anything get in the way of what you want to do.

Ask for Advice

If you're struggling with any aspect of creating content or managing an audience, ask for help and advice from someone who you know does it well. The online community is generally very friendly and helpful. I've asked so many friends for tips along the way, whether it's about choosing the right camera or dealing with admin. If you don't ask for help you won't get it!

Take Inspiration From Others, But Don't Copy Them!

Copying another person's individual style or specific content format is a bad idea for two reasons. It's not original or unique, and your audience will most likely see that, and it's also guaranteed to annoy the person you've copied.

Unplug

This is something that took me a few years to learn, but as with any aspect of your life, it's really important to take some time out every now and again. This will not only help to recharge your (personal) batteries, but it also helps to give you a fresh outlook on your content. If I'm ever struggling for ideas or motivation, taking some time out to reset is the best way to get back into the swing of things.

Be Engaged

The more you engage with your own audience and other content creators over time, the better relationships you'll build with them. This is especially important for cultivating a great bond with your audience, as the ability to interact with someone you watch or follow is what makes the internet so special.

Think Outside the Box

It's easy to see one person achieving success and think that following their lead is the only way to go, but it's also important to stick to your guns and produce content that you love making. If you're not interested in what's in the 'box', then think outside of it and keep making the content you love. The chances are that even if your audience is not as big, they'll be more dedicated and interested and will stick around for longer.

Don't Underestimate the Importance of Admin

Whether it's creating a great thumbnail, taking a few minutes extra to think about the title, or writing a perfectly detailed description for a video, admin can make a huge difference to your video views. You might be making great content, but if you're not packaging it well, it won't reach its maximum potential.

Streamline the Process

You can make your life a lot easier when it comes to promoting your content by using social media management sites like HootSuite or TweetDeck. This allows you to be more efficient and track your progress more easily, giving you time to dedicate to making the content itself.

Get Personal

Another reason why YouTube is so special and so successful is the personal nature of the content. The more effort you make to let your audience get to know you, the stronger a connection you'll build.

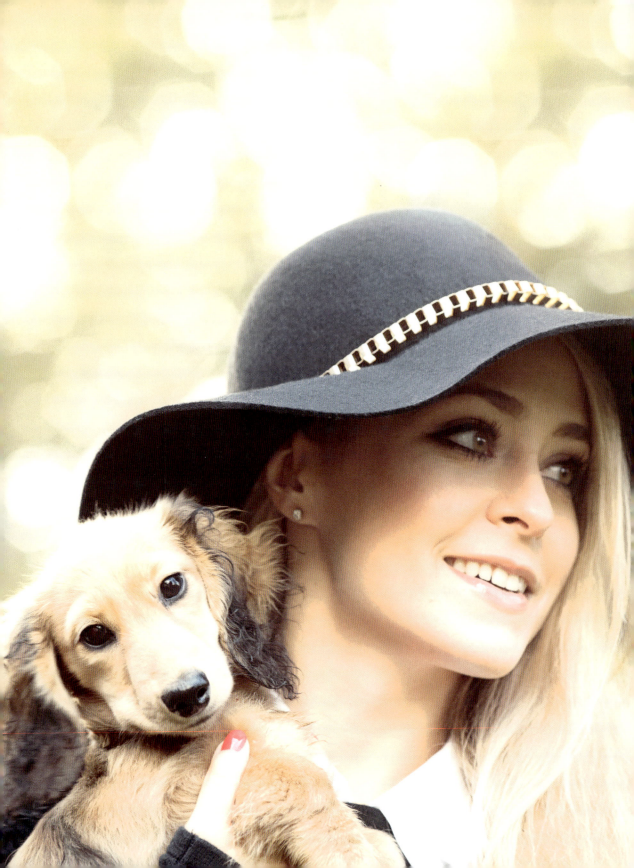

A Note to My Subscribers

I hope you enjoyed this book. I wrote it in the hope that you would walk away feeling just that little bit more confident and inspired. You've helped me so much over the past five years, but especially so with this book. It's been a truly collaborative experience, and I couldn't be more grateful for your comments, feedback, advice and support throughout. As always, I would love to hear from you, about the book or anything else, so please get in touch.

With love,

fleur x

Acknowledgements

Thank you to the wonderful team at Headline who have helped bring this book to life. To my editor Sarah Emsley and her assistant Holly Harris for their advice, suggestions and feedback, thank you for believing in me from the beginning when I said I wanted to write this book alone despite having absolutely no experience. Thank you for your guidance and patience throughout.

To my incredibly talented and hard-working designer Siobhan Hooper, who seemed to know exactly what I was thinking before I told her, thank you for your enthusiasm, cheerfulness and for managing to make this book look even better than I had envisioned. To the wonderful Sally Faye Cotterill (who I have been not-so-secretly stalking online for years), thank you for coming on board to illustrate this book. You are fabulous.

A thousand thank yous to my management team at James Grant, Mary Bekhait and Amy Newman. Few people writing a book about all things glamorous and girly are lucky enough to have a management team far more glamorous than they are looking after the serious stuff! To my literary agent Rory Scarfe, I apologise for you having to work on the girliest book in the world, but thank you for being relentlessly enthusiastic throughout. I couldn't have asked for a better team around me to help make this happen.

To my wonderful husband Mike, thank you for being there for me always. No matter how stressed, grumpy or absent I've been during the process of writing this book, you've always given me unquestioned, unwavering support. I feel so privileged to have you next to me on this journey they call life.

Thank you to my amazing family for understanding my obsession from the very beginning, encouraging me every step of the way and always being there to keep my feet firmly on the ground. I love you all very much.

To my amazing friends. I can't possibly name you all, but you know who you are. Thanks for being there for me and putting up with my strange YouTube ways. Most of you have been there for many years, and I hope you are all there for many more.

Lastly, thank you to my followers. Without your support this book would never have happened. I'm eternally grateful to you all for the love, feedback, suggestions and encouragement you've given me throughout my time on YouTube. You really have changed my life and for that there are no words.